MCQs AND OSCEs IN OPTICS AND REFRACTION

A Bhan

Senior House Officer in Ophthalmology,
Royal Hallamshire Hospital,
Sheffield

VJK Menon

Specialist Registrar in Ophthalmology,
Royal Hallamshire Hospital,
Sheffield

IM Whelehan

Specialist Registrar in Ophthalmology,
Royal Hallamshire Hospital,
Sheffield

J Whittle

Lecturer in Orthoptics,
University Department of Orthoptics and Ophthalmology,
University of Sheffield

BMJ
Books

© BMJ Publishing Group 1999
BMJ Books is an imprint of the BMJ Publishing Group

First published in 1999
by BMJ Books, BMA House, Tavistock Square,
London WC1H 9JR

British Library Cataloguing in Publication Data

A catalogue record for this book is available from the
British Library

ISBN 0 7279 1272 0

Typeset, printed and bound in Great Britain by
Latimer Trend & Company Ltd, Plymouth

Contents

Foreword

To be honest, optics has never been my strong suit. I've often quipped that you could write down the sum total of my knowledge on the subject on a modest sized postcard with ample space remaining for a fairly lengthy address. I well remember the flood of relief I experienced when, as a junior, I read the question paper at my Fellowship examination and realised that, not only was there a dearth of optics questions, but that those that were present I could actually answer!

Like it or not things have changed. The Royal College of Ophthalmologists examination board quite rightly recognise the importance of both theoretical and clinical optics and have devised an examination format which tests both basic knowledge and practical skills. Of course optics is only one part of the Royal College of Ophthalmologists Part II membership examination, the successful candidate must also now prove that he or she has a sound understanding of clinical methodology. The authors have produced this book with the specific aim of helping candidates prepare for the membership examination. It is not a textbook of optics, nor is it meant to be. Used correctly, I'm sure this book will find favour by all readers.

I G Rennie
Professor of Ophthalmology
Royal Hallamshire Hospital
Sheffield

Acknowledgments

We would like to thank the following people for their assistance in preparation of this book: Mary Banks of BMJ Publishing for her patience and encouragement; Chris Mody, Laura Strong, Robin Farr, and Lawrence Brown at the RHH for preparation of the pictorial material; Deborah Parkinson for help with orthoptics; Andrea Sleeth for her help with the manuscript; all the Consultants at the RHH for provision of subject matter; Kanchan Bhan, Girdari Bhan, Dipan Mistry, and Hugh Wyrley-Birch for help with the multiple choice questions; Professor Ian Rennie for the Foreword; and Mr John Talbot, previous chief examiner for Optics, for advice on the manuscript.

Preface

Whilst preparing for the optics and refraction part of the FRCOphth, it became apparent to us that there was a paucity of self testing material to aid revision. Subsequent to our passing the examination, we set about writing multiple choice questions to help future candidates. We then had to take into account the new examination structure of the Part II MRCOphth and accordingly have added a new section containing short questions and cases similar to those in the OSCE section of this exam. Finally we have written a third section which describes in detail practical refraction and other skills which will be helpful in clinical practice as well as in preparing for the exam. The end result is a book with ample subject material to enable a candidate to focus their revision at the level and subject matter necessary for the new examination.

The new examination has four components. The first is a **multiple choice question** paper of 60 stems each with 5 questions. Subject matter will include optics, refraction, and clinical methods. Second is a **refraction practical** lasting one half-hour; during this period the first 15 minutes with the patient will be unsupervised and the remaining 15 minutes will be under observation by the examiners. The third and fourth parts are **OSCEs** (objective structured clinical examinations). The optics OSCE lasts half an hour and the clinical methods OSCE lasts one hour.

An OSCE comprises a series of timed stations where examinees are required to perform clinically orientated tasks, data interpretation, and communication skills. A station will be either observer-based or unobserved, i.e. the candidate submits a written answer. Each station is individually marked according to a predetermined list of objectives for determining competence in a particular skill under test. Stations are standardised and objective in that each candidate undergoes the same assessment under identical conditions.

Both OSCE sections must be passed. The optics OSCE may assess skills such as correct use of a focimeter or keratometer, drawing ray diagrams, or optical calculations may be set. The OSCE format is particularly relevant for use in the clinical methods examination. Pupil examination, use of the slit lamp, ocular movements and measuring the angle of strabismus are examples of clinical skills likely to be assessed in front of an examiner. Written stations may include interpretation of fluorescein angiograms, visual fields or CT scans. The syllabus, as published by the Royal College of Ophthalmologists, for these two sections is listed below. In the OSCE section of this book we have given examples of OSCE type questions. Obviously it is not possible to examine clinical skills in a book format, instead clinical pictures have been used as a basis for these questions. In preparation for this examination we recommend that you practise clinical examination in front of teachers and peers until you become proficient at eliciting clinical signs efficiently and accurately.

In the OSCE part of the examination points will be allotted to each part of a question. We have not allotted points, instead we have expanded the answer with explanations where not specifically asked for in the question. At the time of writing this book OSCEs have only recently been introduced in the last two sittings of the Part II MRCOphth, it is therefore an evolving examination. This section of the book is written as a guide to prospective candidates of what might be expected from the new format and is not necessarily a true representation of the new examination. This section of the book is therefore best used to help direct further study in preparation for this examination.

To help preparation for the examination we have included a brief reading list. Coverage of the relevant sections in these texts should give ample knowledge for the examination. Practice of the multiple choice and OSCE questions will help guide preparation also. Refraction is a very important part of the examination and we strongly encourage candidates to gain as much experience as possible in this aspect as this component carries the most importance and failing it results in failure of the whole examination.

Although the details in the book have been checked very thoroughly and as far as we know are correct, it is possible that occasional errors may have been made and we apologise if that is the case.

It would be advisable for candidates to ensure that the current system of examination, listed above, has not changed. Any suggestions for improvement in this book would be welcomed.

Syllabus for the OSCE section of the Royal College of Ophthalmologists Part II Membership Examination

OSCE – Optics

Focimetry
Lens identification
Lens transposition
Retinoscopy (trial eye)
Keratometry
Corneal topography
Calculations – focal length
             – lens decentration

Ray diagrams
Prescribing for children
Contact lens fitting
Inter-pupillary distance

OSCE – Clinical Methods

Pupil reactions
Visual field testing/interpretation
Ocular motility (including ptosis, nystagmus, cover test, and prism bar)
Fluorescein angiography
Exophthalmometry
CT/MR scans
X-rays of skull and orbit
Ultrasound scans (A- and B-scans)
Electrodiagnostics
Ophthalmoscopy – direct and indirect
Use of slit lamp and lenses
Hess charts/orthoptic reports

Recommended texts

Elkington AR, Frank HJ. *Clinical Optics*, 2nd edition. Oxford: Blackwell Scientific, 1991.
Abrams D (ed). *Duke-Elder's Practice of Refraction*, 10th edition. Edinburgh: Churchill Livingstone, 1993.
Kanski JJ. *Clinical Ophthalmology*, 4th edition. Oxford: Butterworth Heinemann, 1999.
American Academy of Ophthalmology. *Basic and Clinical Science Course*. San Francisco: American Academy of Ophthalmology, 1997–8.
   Section 3: *Optics, Refraction and Contact Lenses*.
   Section 5: *Neuro-ophthalmology*.
   Section 6: *Pediatric Ophthalmology and Strabismus*.
Mein J, Trimble R. *Diagnosis and Management of Ocular Motility Disorders*, 2nd edition. Oxford: Blackwell Scientific, 1991.

A Bhan
I M Whelehan

Part One

MCQs

Physical optics

Questions

1 The wavelength of light:

   a Does not change as it passes through a denser medium. F
   b Is inversely proportional to its frequency.
   c Is the distance between two symmetrical parts of the wave.
   d Is the same as its amplitude.
   e Is equal to a cycle in a waveform

2 Light

The following are true:

   a Shorter wavelengths have greater energy.
   b The frequency of light changes when it passes from one medium to the next.
   c Two waves in phase with one another result in constructive interference if they travel in the same direction.
   d Incoherent light is composed of waves that are out of phase.
   e The photoreceptors of the eye are only sensitive to wavelength between 400 and 780 nm.

3 Polarisation

The following are true:

   a Polarised light consists of waves which are parallel to each other.
   b Polarising glasses are used to dissociate eyes.
   c Polarised light is used to examine optic lenses.
   d Light incident on a water surface may be polarised.
   e Slit lamps use polarised light.

4 Interference

The following are true:

a   The clarity of the cornea is due to constructive interference.
b   Anti-reflection films work on the principle of destructive interference.
c   Waves of equal amplitude and out of phase by half a cycle cancel each other out.
d   Phase difference of less than half a cycle results in a wave of intermediate amplitude.
e   Interference filters transmit only one wavelength.

5 Stereopsis

The following are true:

a   Stereopsis is the least horizontal disparity which evokes a perception of depth.
b   Normal stereoacuity is approximately 60 minutes of a degree.
c   Stereopsis of 250 seconds excludes significant amblyopia.
d   Stereoacuity is tested for each eye individually.
e   Stereoacuity is maximum when the image falls on the maculae.

6 The following are true:

a   The TNO test requires polarising glasses.
b   The Frisby test does not require glasses to be worn.
c   The Lang stereotest does not offer monocular clues.
d   The Wirt fly test is done with polarising glasses.
e   The viewing distance may be adjusted while assessing with the Frisby test.

7 The following are true:

a   An anaglyph is a stereogram.
b   Red–green spectacles are used to view a vectograph.
c   The Titmus test is an example of a vectograph.
d   A vectograph is based on the principle of polarisation.
e   The image seen through the red–green glasses in a TNO test appears yellow.

8 Visual acuity

The following are true:

a The resolving power of the eye is the smallest angle of separation between two points which forms two discernible images on the retina.

b At 1 minute of a degree, in the normal eye, two retinal images are separated by at least one non-stimulated cone.

c If a patient reads the top letter of the Snellen chart at 60 m, he has a visual acuity of at least 6/60.

d To recognise a letter, the eye must have a limit of resolution of one minute of a degree.

e A visual acuity of 6/60 is equal to 20/200.

9 Diffraction:

a Is the main source of image imperfection in the eye.

b Is most marked with small apertures.

c Through a circular aperture produces a dark central zone.

d Is based on the principle of interference.

e Through a circular aperture produces alternate dark and light bands surrounding the Airy disc.

10 Photometry

The following are true:

a Photometry is a qualitative measure of light.

b The human eye is most sensitive to yellow–green light.

c The old unit "candle" is based on the standard wax candle.

d The terms "candela" and the "candle" are interchangeable.

e Illumination of a surface is directly related to the distance of the surface from the light source.

11 Stereoacuity tests include:

a Frisby test

b TNO test

c Titmus test

d Lang test

e Wirt fly test

12 The following are true:

    a Luminance is the amount of light arriving at a surface.
    b Luminous flux is the amount of light emitted in a given direction by a source.
    c Luminous flux is measured in candelas.
    d Illumination of a surface is dependent on the angle of incident light.
    e The Lambert system assumes the reflecting surface to be a perfect diffuser.

13 Regarding the lumen:

    a The lumen is the unit of measurement of luminous flux.
    b Lumen/ft^2 is a measure of surface illumination.
    c 1 lumen/steridian = 1 Lambert.
    d 1 lumen/ft^2 = 1 ft-Lambert.
    e It is the unit of measure of luminance.

14 Regarding laser design and resonance chambers

Lasers:

    a Use the principle of constructive interference.
    b Contain plane mirrors.
    c Produce polychromatic and coherent light.
    d Their length is a multiple of the wavelength of the emitted light.
    e Have an aperture to allow emission of light.

15 Ophthalmic lasers

The following are true:

    a The argon laser produces a yellow–red light.
    b The HeNe gas laser is used as an aiming beam.
    c Semiconductor lasers have the advantage of being small and portable.
    d Q-switched lasers obtain very high levels of population inversion.
    e Continuous wave laser light may be used with the slit lamp microscope by means of prisms.

16 The Nd–YAG laser:

    a Is a noble gas laser.

    b Uses the photochemical effect to perform peripheral iridotomies.

    c Produces blue–green light.

    d May be used to produce mode locked pulses.

    e Should be used with a focusing contact lens when performing a peripheral iridotomy.

17 Regarding photo-toxicity:

    a UV light can cause retinal toxicity.

    b UV light does not cause endothelial damage acutely.

    c Infra-red radiation can cause eclipse burns.

    d The natural lens absorbs harmful UV light between 400 and 780 nm.

    e PMMA lenses mostly absorb UV light below 320 nm.

18 Excimer lasers

The following are true:

    a The term excimer laser is derived from "excited dimer".

    b Excimer lasers contain noble gas-halogen combinations.

    c The Excimer XECI laser emits UV light.

    d Excimer lasers are used to photoablate the cornea to change its refractive power.

    e Excimer lasers are known to cause endothelial decompensation.

19 Retinal pigment absorption

The following are true:

    a The main ocular pigments are haemoglobin, melanin and xanthophyll.

    b Argon blue is highly absorbed by xanthophyll.

    c Xanthophyll absorbs krypton well.

    d Krypton laser is the treatment of choice for macula laser therapy.

    e The xenon laser is usually used for panretinal photocoagulation.

Physical optics

Answers

1 a **False.** The wavelength of light reduces as it passes through a denser medium.
$\lambda v \, / \, \lambda m = n_{\mathrm{m}}$, where λv = wavelength of light in a vacuum, λm = wavelength of light in a medium of refractive index n_{m}.

b **True.**

c **True.**

d **False.** Amplitude is the maximum displacement of an imaginary particle on the wave from the base line.

e **True.**

2 a **True.** $E = hc \, / \, \lambda$, where E = energy per photon, h = Planck's constant 6.62×10^{-34} joule/sec, c = speed of light in a vacuum, λ = wavelength.

b **False.** Frequency does not change, but wavelength does.

c **True.** The resultant wave will be the summation of the two, i.e. constructive interference.

d **True.**

e **False.** They are also sensitive to wavelengths between 350 and 400 nm (UV–A).

3 a **True.** All wave motions in polarised light vibrate in the same plane and are parallel to each other.

b **True.** As in the Titmus test.

c **True.**

d **True.** If the angle of incidence is equal to the polarising angle of the surface, polarisation occurs.

e **True.**

4 a **False.** Destructive interference occurs due to the arrangement of collagen bundles within the stroma.
  b **True.** The anti-reflection coating is a thin layer of transparent material applied to the lens surface. Light rays reflected from the superficial and deep surfaces of the layer eliminate each other (i.e. destructive interference).
  c **True.** This is destructive interference.
  d **True.** The resultant wave is of intermediate amplitude and phase.
  e **True.** Interference filters are designed so that successive rays transmitted through are exactly in phase. Therefore, only one wavelength of light is transmitted by an interference filter.

5 a **True.**
  b **False.** Normal stereoacuity is 60 *seconds* of arc or better.
  c **True.**
  d **False.** Stereopsis is a function of binocular vision and cannot be assessed for an individual eye.
  e **True.**

6 a **False.** Red–green glasses are worn.
  b **True.**
  c **False.** If the test card is not held parallel to the subject's face, uniocular clues will be found.
  d **True.**
  e **True.**

7 a **True.** In an anaglyph, two disparate views are printed in red and green.
  b **False.** Red–green spectacles are used to view an anaglyph, e.g. TNO test.
  c **True.**
  d **True.**
  e **False.** The eye looking through the red filter at the green picture sees only a black image and that looking through the green filter sees the red picture as black. The two views are fused for a stereoscopic effect.

8 a   True.

  b   True.

  c   False. The numerator indicates the distance at which the letter is read. Thus, the visual acuity would be 60/60. In practice, vision is first tested at 6 m and the patient is moved closer, i.e. 5 m, 4 m etc., if they cannot read the chart at 6 m.

  d   True.

  e   True. The American system uses the latter system, where 20 implies 20 feet (which equals 6 m).

9 a   True. Diffraction is most marked when the pupil is small.

  b   True. It occurs in optical lenses, optical instruments and the eye.

  c   False. A bright central zone is produced, known as the Airy disc.

  d   True. Interference between the primary and secondary waves is responsible for diffraction.

  e   True. Dark bands receive light from the secondary waves while the light bands receive light from both primary and secondary waves.

10 a   False. Photometry is a *quantitative* measurement of light.

  b   True.

  c   True.

  d   True.

  e   False. Illumination is *inversely* related to the distance of the surface from the light source – Cosine law.

$$E = \frac{I \cos i}{d^2}$$

11 a   True. The Frisby consists of three plastic plates of different thickness with four squares on each. One square in each plate has a hidden pattern. It can be used to give a disparity range of 600 to 15 seconds of an arc.

  b   True. The TNO test consists of two disparate views printed in red and green. When viewed through a red–green spectacle the two views are fused to give a stereoscopic effect. It tests disparities between 480 to 15 seconds.

  c   True. The Titmus test uses a polarising visor to view the composite picture. It tests stereoacuity in the range of 300 to 40 seconds of an arc.

  d   True. In the Lang test the targets are fine vertical lines which are seen alternately by each eye through cylindrical lenses. Disparities between 1200 to 550 seconds of an arc may be tested.

  e   True. The Wirt fly test is the largest target in the Titmus test.

12 a **False.** Luminance is the measure of light reflected or emitted by a surface.

b **False.** Luminous intensity of a source measures light emitted in a given direction.

c **False.** Candela is the unit of measurement of luminous intensity.

d **True.**

$$\frac{E = I \cos i}{d^2},$$

where E = illumination, I = luminous intensity, i = angle of incidence, d = distance source and surface.

e **True.**

13 a **True.**

b **True.**

c **False.** 1 lumen/steridian = 1 candela.

d **True.**

e **False.** The lumen is the unit of luminous flux.

14 a **True.** Here the light traversing the resonance chamber is exactly in phase and reinforces itself.

b **True.**

c **False.** Produce *monochromatic* light.

d **True.** This enables resonance to occur.

e **True.**

15 a **False.** The argon laser produces a blue–green light of wavelength 488–515 nm, which is absorbed by all ocular pigments.

b **True.** It produces a red beam which is used as an aiming beam for lasers with output outside the visible spectrum.

c **True.** Semiconductor or diode lasers are also relatively cheap and very efficient. They must be used with an aiming beam as their output is in the range 790–950 nm.

d **True.** Q-switched laser involves short single laser pulses of very high power.

e **True.** Continuous wave laser light may be used with the slit lamp either with prisms, as in the Nd–YAG laser, or with a fibreoptic system.

16 a False. The Nd–YAG laser is a crystal laser.

   b False. The Nd–YAG laser uses the *ionising* effect to perform peripheral iridotomies. Here the target area is ionised into a plasma which disrupts adjacent tissue.

   c False. The Nd–YAG produces light of wavelength 1.065 micrometres, which is infra-red and hence invisible to the eye.

   d True. The Nd–YAG is a continuous wave laser which may be used to produce mode locked pulses.

   e True. The contact lens helps to concentrate the energy delivered to the iris, and absorbs heat, reducing the risk of corneal damage.

17 a True.

   b False. UV light *may* cause endothelial damage acutely.

   c True.

   d False. The natural lens absorbs harmful UV–A light between 400 and 350 nm.

   e True. Hence UV–A light of wavelength 320–400 nm may cause retinal damage if PMMA lenses are used.

18 a True. The dimer is bound when excited but decays to give its component atoms, producing very high energy photons which allow photoablation of the corneal surface without damage to the remaining tissue.

   b True. For example, the xenon–chloride and argon–fluoride excimer lasers.

   c True.

   d True.

   e False. The long term effects of excimer laser therapy are unknown.

19 a True.

   b True. This is the reason why argon blue is not recommended for macula photocoagulation.

   c False. Krypton red is well absorbed by melanin but poorly absorbed by xanthophyll and haemoglobin.

   d True. Krypton is poorly absorbed by xanthophyll so lesions within the foveal arcades may be treated with minimal damage to the neural retina. Xenon has a similar absorption pattern but the spot size is too large for it to be used close to the fovea.

   e True. Its main advantage is that it can treat large areas of retina quickly – this is useful for panretinal photocoagulation and certain ocular tumours.

Geometric optics

Questions

1 Reflection

The following are true:

a The angle of incidence equals the angle of reflection.
b An image formed by a plane mirror is laterally inverted and real.
c A concave mirror always forms a virtual image.
d A convex mirror always forms an erect image.
e Convex mirrors give a large field of view.

2 Refraction

The following are true:

a The angle of incidence is equal to the angle of refraction.
b When light passes through a more dense medium it is deviated towards the normal.
c The refractive index of a material is inversely proportional to the velocity of light in that medium.
d When the angle of incidence exceeds the critical angle total internal reflection occurs.
e Total internal reflection occurs in the peripheral retina.

3 Refraction of light

The following are true:

a The ratio of the velocity of light in a vacuum and in another medium is the absolute refractive index of the medium.
b Crown glass has a higher refractive index than flint glass.

13

    c The refractometer determines the absolute refractive index of any material.

    d The teaching mirror of an indirect ophthalmoscope employs the property of refraction.

    e Light waves refracted by a surface undergo a change of frequency.

4 Reflection

The following are true:

    a The first law of reflection states that the incident, reflected, and normal rays all lie in the same plane.

    b The second law of reflection states that the angles of incidence and refraction are related to the refractive index of the refracting medium.

    c Reflection by a plane mirror gives a virtual, laterally and vertically inverted, image.

    d If a plane mirror is rotated through angle alpha (α), the angle through which the reflected rays are deviated is 2α.

    e Convex mirrors always produce a virtual diminished image.

5 Reflection

The following are true:

    a Diffuse reflection describes reflection by an irregular surface.

    b The image formed of an object by reflection from a plane surface is always as far behind the reflecting surface as the object is in front of it.

    c A concave mirror adds positive vergence to incident light.

    d Real images can be captured on a screen.

    e A plane mirror adds negative vergence to incident light.

6 For a concave mirror with the object between the centre of curvature (C) and the principal focus, the image is:

    a Real.

    b Upright.

    c Magnified.

    d Outside C.

    e Diminished.

7 The image formed by a convex mirror is:

a Real.
b Upright.
c The same size as the object.
d Located between F and the mirror.
e Between F and C.

8 Reflection

The following are true:

a In prism binoculars prisms are used as reflectors.
b The transmission of laser light from the laser tube to the slit lamp is based on the principle of total internal reflection.
c Significant amounts of light are lost by reflection as it transmits through the length of a fibreoptic cable.
d Bending a fibreoptic cable impairs its efficiency.
e The largest of the three mirrors in a Goldmann-triple mirror lens helps visualise the angle of the anterior chamber.

9 For a concave mirror with an object outside the centre of curvature C, the image is:

a Real.
b Upright.
c Diminished.
d Lying between F and the mirror.
e Lying between C and the principal focus.

10 Thin lenses

The following are true:

a Lens power calculation incorporates an adjustment for lens thickness.
b The nodal point is the point at which the principal plane and principal axis intersect.
c Rays through the optical centre are undeviated.
d The first principal focus is the point to which parallel light rays converge following refraction by a spherical lens.
e Vergence power is proportional to focal length.

15

11 Lens decentration

The following are true:

a Decentration of a lens is use of a non-axial portion of the lens to gain a prismatic effect.
b Decentration can cause a jack-in-the-box effect.
c Prismatic effect may be calculated using lens power in dioptres and decentration in centimetres.
d The prismatic effect of the downward decentration of a $+12$ dioptre lens by 3 mm is 3.6 base up.
e Upward decentration of a -6 dioptre lens by 5 mm causes a 3 dioptre base out prismatic effect.

12 In optical terms, a lens can be considered thin under the following circumstances:

a If its thickness is small in relation to its focal length, and the object and image distances.
b If its power is less than 5 DS.
c If the front and back surfaces are of equal curvature.
d If its thickness is less than 3 mm.
e If its refractive index is less than 1.7.

13 Considering thin lenses:

a If two thin lenses, of power $+2$ DS and -1 DS are held in contact with each other the focal length of the combination of lenses will be 1 m.
b If two thin lenses, of power $+2$ DS and -1 DS are separated by a distance of 0.5 m, the combination of lenses would make a Galilean telescope.
c If an object is located 0.50 m from a thin lens of power $+4$ DS, a real image will be formed 0.20 m from the lens.
d If an object is located 0.125 m from a thin lens of power $+4$ DS, a virtual image will be formed at a distance of -0.25 m from the lens.
e If an object is placed 0.20 m from a thin lens of power $+2$ DS, an image is formed 0.40 m from the lens.

14 Regarding prisms:

   a The apical angle of a crown glass prism is twice the angle of deviation.
   b The image is displaced towards the base of the prism.
   c The position of minimum deviation is the Prentice position.
   d The Prentice position requires one surface of the prism to be perpendicular to the incident ray.
   e The Prentice position is used most commonly in ophthalmic assessment.

15 Prisms

The following are true:

   a The "centrad" measures the image displacement along an arc 1 cm from a prism.
   b The "centrad" and "prism dioptre" produce the same angle of deviation.
   c Prisms may be used in the assessment of simulated blindness.
   d Prisms are used preoperatively to assess the likelihood of diplopia after squint surgery in adults.
   e The Maddox rod is comprised of high powered prisms.

16 Prisms are used in the:

   a Panfundoscope.
   b Keratometer.
   c Applanation tonometer.
   d Slit lamp.
   e Direct ophthalmoscope.

17 Regarding prisms:

   a A 10Δ base out prism with an 8Δ base out prism on top gives a total power of 18Δ base out, if the prisms are not considered to be thin.
   b A 6Δ prism has a refracting angle of 12 degrees, if made from glass with refractive index 1.5.

    c A prism which deviates light through 14 degrees has a power of 7Δ, assuming its refractive index is 1.5.

    d A 1Δ prism produces a linear apparent displacement of 1 m of an object at 1 cm.

    e Centrads measure angular deviation.

18 Fresnel prisms:

    a Are lightweight.

    b May reduce visual acuity.

    c Consist of a plastic sheet of tiny prisms, the overall effect being equal to a single large prism.

    d May be incorporated permanently into glasses.

    e Consist of a sheet of tiny parallel prisms of increasing size.

19 Regarding therapeutic use of prisms:

    a Permanent prisms may be incorporated into spectacles by lens decentration.

    b To correct a 20Δ exotropia, 10Δ base in prisms should be used bilaterally.

    c To correct a 10Δ right hypotropia requires a 5Δ base down prism in front of the right eye and a 5Δ base up prism in front of the left eye.

    d The apex of the prism should be placed towards the direction of deviation of the eye.

    e Convergence excess may be corrected with base out prisms.

20 Regarding types of prisms:

    a A Porro prism is right-angled.

    b A Dove prism laterally and vertically inverts the image.

    c Porro prisms are used to shorten ophthalmic instruments.

    d Prisms may totally internally reflect light.

    e The Goldmann applanation tonometer contains 2 prisms.

21 Regarding refraction of light:

  a Light entering a more dense medium is deviated towards the refracting interface.

  b The absolute refractive index of a substance equals the velocity of light in a vacuum divided by the velocity of light in the substance.

  c The incident ray, the refracted ray, and the normal are all perpendicular to each other.

  d Snell's law states that

$$n = \frac{\text{Sin } i}{r}$$

  e Light passing through a pane of glass is laterally displaced and parallel to the incident ray.

22 Regarding refraction at a curved interface:

  a Light passing across a curved interface obeys Snell's law.

  b Light entering a convexly curved surface of greater refractive index is converged.

  c The surface power of a curved interface =

$$\frac{n_1 - n_2}{r}$$

  where r = the radius of curvature of the surface in metres, and n_1 and n_2 are the refractive indices on either side of the interface.

  d The surface power is positive for a diverging surface and negative for a converging surface.

  e The anterior corneal surface is a converging surface accounting for most of the eye's refractive power.

23 Spectacles

The following are true:

  a A toric surface is curved in both its horizontal and vertical meridians.

  b The principal meridians are the meridians of maximum curvature.

  c In ophthalmic lenses, these meridians are at right-angles to each other.

  d A toric lens is a sphero-cylindrical lens.

  e Jackson's cross cylinder is used to define the direction but not the strength of the cylinder.

19

24 The cross cylinder:

    a Is a sphero-cylindrical lens.

    b The handle is mounted at 90 degrees to the axes of the cylinder.

    c The axes marked on the lens are axes of no power of individual cylinders.

    d A 0.5 DC cylinder is used to check the trial cylinder in a patient with good vision.

    e A cross cylinder of 1 DC is equivalent to

$$\frac{-0.50\,\text{DS}}{+1.0\,\text{DC}}$$

25 Regarding apparent depth and the critical angle:

    a Apparent depth is seen when objects in a less optically dense medium appear more superficial than they actually are.

    b Apparent depth is due to refraction of emerging rays creating a real image.

    c Apparent depth is important in intra-ocular surgery.

    d Incident rays of greater angle than the critical angle undergo total internal reflection.

    e Total internal reflection occurs with structures in the peripheral retina.

26 Regarding gonioscopes:

    a Gonioscope contact lenses overcome total internal reflection by neutralising the cornea:air refracting surface.

    b Gonioscopes contain a plane mirror.

    c The Zeiss goniolens is used with a viscous coupling fluid.

    d The Goldmann gonioscope has a curvature steeper than the cornea.

    e The Koeppe is an indirect goniolens.

27 Dispersion

The following are true:

    a Dispersion occurs when white light is refracted at an optical interface.

    b Short wavelength light is deviated less than long wavelength light.

    c The angle between red and blue dispersed light relates to the dispersive power of the medium.

    d Dispersion is the underlying principle behind chromatic aberration.

    e Dispersion is the underlying principle behind the duochrome test.

28 Chromatic aberration

The following are true:

a Chromatic aberration accounts for 3 dioptres of aberration in the human eye.
b The higher the refractive index of a material the higher its dispersive power.
c The duochrome test is sensitive to a difference of 0.25 dioptres.
d Shorter wavelengths are deviated more at an optical interface.
e The duochrome test is always inaccurate in a protanope.

29 Spherical aberration:

a Is reduced by the use of stops.
b Is most through the paraxial zone of a lens.
c Increases with a dilated pupil.
d Can be reduced with doublets.
e Is more with a planoconvex than a biconvex lens.

30 Aberrations

The following are true:

a Oblique astigmatism is based on the principle of Sturm's Conoid.
b Oblique astigmatism in the eye is reduced to a certain extent by the poor resolution of images in the peripheral retina.
c Coma is a form of oblique astigmatism.
d Coma is corrected by stops.
e Retinal curvature partially compensates for field curvature in the eye.

31 The following are true:

a Aplanatic lenses correct chromatic aberrations.
b Doublets consist of a principal lens and a weaker lens of opposite power.
c Doublets counter spherical and chromatic aberration.
d Prismatic effect of a spherical lens is least at its optical centre.
e Image distortion is due to the prismatic effect at the periphery of the lens.

32 The following are true:

  a Pin cushion distortion is typical in high power concave lenses.
  b The jack-in-the-box effect is explained on the basis of barrel distortion.
  c Curvature of field is an aberration caused by curvature of the lens.
  d Curvature of field is influenced by the refractive index of the lens.
  e Curvature of field is present even when spherical and chromatic aberrations have been eliminated.

33 The Geneva lens measure:

  a Measures the surface powers of a lens.
  b Uses the principle that the total power of a thin lens equals the sum of its surface powers.
  c Is calibrated for flint glass.
  d Consists of a focusing system and an observation system.
  e Is the most commonly used method of estimating lens power.

34 A prescription of $+3.50\,\text{DS}/+2.50\,\text{DC} \times 60$ is equivalent to:

  a $+3.50\,\text{DS}/-2.50\,\text{DC} \times 60$
  b $+3.50\,\text{DS}/-2.50\,\text{DC} \times 30$
  c $-3.50\,\text{DS}/-2.50\,\text{DC} \times 120$
  d $+6.00\,\text{DS}/-2.50\,\text{DC} \times 150$
  e $+1.00\,\text{DS}/-2.50\,\text{DC} \times 120$

35 A prescription of $+1.00\,\text{DS}/-3.00\,\text{DC} \times 90$ is equivalent to:

  a $+4.00\,\text{DS}/-3.00\,\text{DC} \times 90$
  b $-2.00\,\text{DS}/+3.00\,\text{DC} \times 180$
  c $-2.00\,\text{DS}/+3.00\,\text{DC} \times 90$
  d $+4.00\,\text{DS}/+3.00\,\text{DC} \times 180$
  e $-2.00\,\text{DS}/-3.00\,\text{DC} \times 180$

36 A prescription of $-4.00\,\mathrm{DS}/+1.00\,\mathrm{DC} \times 95$ is equivalent to:

   a $-5.00\,\mathrm{DS}/-1.00\,\mathrm{DC} \times 85$
   b $-3.00\,\mathrm{DS}/-1.00\,\mathrm{DC} \times 95$
   c $-5.00\,\mathrm{DS}/-1.00\,\mathrm{DC} \times 5$
   d $-3.00\,\mathrm{DS}/-1.00\,\mathrm{DC} \times 5$
   e $-3.00\,\mathrm{DS}/+1.00\,\mathrm{DC} \times 5$

37 The toric transposition of $+2.00\,\mathrm{DS}/+1.00\,\mathrm{DC} \times 90$ to the base curve $+6$ is:

   a $$\frac{+9.00}{-6.00\,\mathrm{DC} \times 90/-7.00\,\mathrm{DC} \times 180}$$

   b $$\frac{+6.00\,\mathrm{DC} \times 180/+7.00\,\mathrm{DC} \times 90}{-4.00}$$

   c $$\frac{+7.00\,\mathrm{DS}}{-6.00\,\mathrm{DC} \times 90/-7.00\,\mathrm{DC} \times 180}$$

   d $$\frac{+4.00\,\mathrm{DS}}{-6.00\,\mathrm{DC} \times 90/-7.00\,\mathrm{DC} \times 180}$$

   e $$\frac{+7.00\,\mathrm{DS}}{-6.00\,\mathrm{DC} \times 180/+7.00\,\mathrm{DC} \times 90}$$

38 The toric transposition of $+1.00\,\mathrm{DS}/+3.00\,\mathrm{DC} \times 90$ to the base curve -6.00 is:

   a $$\frac{+6.00\,\mathrm{DC} \times 180/+9.00\,\mathrm{DC} \times 90}{-13.00\,\mathrm{DS}}$$

   b $$\frac{+6.00\,\mathrm{DS}}{-5.00\,\mathrm{DC} \times 90/-8.00\,\mathrm{DC} \times 180}$$

   c $$\frac{+7.00\,\mathrm{DC} \times 180/+10.00\,\mathrm{DC} \times 90}{-6.00\,\mathrm{DS}}$$

   d $$\frac{+6.00\,\mathrm{DC} \times 180/+9.00\,\mathrm{DC} \times 90}{-5.00\,\mathrm{DS}}$$

   e $$\frac{+6.00\,\mathrm{DS}}{-2.00\,\mathrm{DC} \times 90/-5.00\,\mathrm{DC} \times 180}$$

39 A prescription of $+3.00\,\text{DS}/+1.00\,\text{DC} \times 20$ is equivalent to:

   a $+4.00\,\text{DS}/-1.00\,\text{DC} \times 70$
   b $+2.00\,\text{DS}/+2.00\,\text{DC} \times 20$
   c $+5.00\,\text{DS}/-1.00\,\text{DC} \times 20$
   d $+4.00\,\text{DS}/-1.00\,\text{DC} \times 110$
   e $+4.00\,\text{DS}/-1.00\,\text{DC} \times 20$

40 A prescription of $-1.00\,\text{DS}/+0.50\,\text{DC} \times 85$ is equivalent to:

   a $+1.00\,\text{DS}/-0.50\,\text{DC} \times 175$
   b $-0.50\,\text{DS}/+0.50\,\text{DC} \times 85$
   c $-0.50\,\text{DS}/-0.50\,\text{DC} \times 175$
   d $-0.50\,\text{DS}/-0.50\,\text{DC} \times 5$
   e $-1.00\,\text{DS}/-0.50\,\text{DC} \times 5$

41 $-2.25\,\text{DS}/+3.00\,\text{DC} \times 140$ is equivalent to:

   a $+0.75\,\text{DS}/-3.00\,\text{DC} \times 50$
   b $+0.75\,\text{DS}/-3.00\,\text{DC} \times 40$
   c $+3.00\,\text{DS}/-2.25\,\text{DC} \times 40$
   d $+3.00\,\text{DS}/-2.25\,\text{DC} \times 50$
   e $+0.75\,\text{DS}/-3.00\,\text{DC} \times 140$

42 The prescription $-1.00\,\text{DS}/-1.00\,\text{DC} \times 180$ is equivalent to:

   a $-2.00\,\text{DS}$
   b $-2.00\,\text{DS}/-1.00\,\text{DC} \times 90$
   c $-2.00\,\text{DS}/+1.00\,\text{DC} \times 90$
   d $-2.00\,\text{DS}/+1.00\,\text{DC} \times 180$
   e $-1.00\,\text{DS}/+2.00\,\text{DC} \times 90$

43 The prescription $-1.00\,\text{DS}/+1.00\,\text{DC} \times 90$ is equivalent to:

   a $+1.00\,\text{DS}/-1.00\,\text{DC} \times 90$
   b $+1.00\,\text{DS}/-1.00\,\text{DC} \times 180$
   c $\text{Plano}/-1.00\,\text{DC} \times 180$
   d $-2.00\,\text{DS}/+3.00\,\text{DC} \times 180$
   e $+2.00\,\text{DS}/-3.00\,\text{DC} \times 180$

44 The toric transposition of $+3.00\,\text{DS}/+1.00\,\text{DC} \times 20$ to the base curve $-2.00\,\text{D}$ is:

a
$$\frac{+5.00\,\text{DS}}{-2.00\,\text{DC} \times 10/+3.00\,\text{DC} \times 110}$$

b
$$\frac{-6.00\,\text{DS}}{-2.00\,\text{DC} \times 20/+1.00\,\text{DC} \times 20}$$

c
$$\frac{+6.00\,\text{DS}}{-2.00\,\text{DC} \times 20/-3.00\,\text{DC} \times 110}$$

d
$$\frac{+3.00\,\text{DS}}{-2.00\,\text{DC} \times 20/+1.00\,\text{DC} \times 110}$$

e
$$\frac{+3.00\,\text{DS}}{-2.00\,\text{DC} \times 110/+1.00\,\text{DC} \times 20}$$

45 The toric transposition of the prescription $-1.00\,\text{DS}/-0.50\,\text{DC} \times 80$ to the base curve $+2.00\,\text{D}$ is:

a
$$\frac{-3.50\,\text{DS}}{+2.00\,\text{DC} \times 80/+2.50\,\text{DC} \times 70}$$

b
$$\frac{-3.50\,\text{DS}}{+2.50\,\text{DC} \times 80/+2.00\,\text{DC} \times 170}$$

c
$$\frac{-3.50\,\text{DS}}{+2.00\,\text{DC} \times 80/-0.50\,\text{DC} \times 10}$$

d
$$\frac{-3.50\,\text{DS}}{-2.00\,\text{DC} \times 170/-0.05\,\text{DC} \times 80}$$

e
$$\frac{+1.00\,\text{DS}}{+2.00\,\text{DC} \times 80/+2.50\,\text{DC} \times 170}$$

25

46 The toric transposition of the prescription $-1.00\,\text{DS}/+1.00\,\text{DC}\ \times$ 90 to the base curve $-2.00\,\text{D}$ is:

a
$$\frac{-1.00\,\text{DS}}{-2.00\,\text{DC} \times 180/+1.00\,\text{DC} \times 90}$$

b
$$\frac{-1.00\,\text{DS}}{-2.00\,\text{DC} \times 90/+1.00\,\text{DC} \times 180}$$

c
$$\frac{+2.00\,\text{DS}}{-2.00\,\text{DC} \times 90/+1.00\,\text{DC} \times 180}$$

d
$$\frac{+2.00\,\text{DS}}{-2.00\,\text{DC} \times 90/-3.00\,\text{DC} \times 180}$$

e
$$\frac{+1.00\,\text{DS}}{-2.00\,\text{DC} \times 90/+3.00\,\text{DC} \times 180}$$

47 The toric transposition of the prescription $-1.00\,\text{DS}/-1.00\,\text{DC}\ \times$ 180 to the base curve $+2.00\,\text{D}$ is:

a
$$\frac{+0.00}{+2.00\,\text{DC} \times 180/+3.00\,\text{DC} \times 90}$$

b
$$\frac{+4.00\,\text{DS}}{+2.00\,\text{DC} \times 180/-1.00\,\text{DC} \times 90}$$

c
$$\frac{-4.00\,\text{DS}}{+2.00\,\text{DC} \times 180/+3.00\,\text{DC} \times 90}$$

d
$$\frac{-4.00\,\text{DS}}{+2.00\,\text{DC} \times 180/-1.00\,\text{DC} \times 90}$$

e
$$\frac{+1.00\,\text{DS}}{+2.00\,\text{DC} \times 180/+3.00\,\text{DC} \times 90}$$

48 The toric transposition of the prescription $-0.25\,\text{DS}/+3.00\,\text{DC} \times 140$ to the base curve $-1.00\,\text{D}$ is:

a
$$\frac{+1.75\,\text{DS}}{-1.00\,\text{DC} \times 140/-4.00\,\text{DC} \times 50}$$

b
$$\frac{-3.25\,\text{DS}}{-1.00\,\text{DC} \times 140/-4.00\,\text{DC} \times 50}$$

c
$$\frac{-3.25\,\text{DS}}{-1.00\,\text{DC} \times 140/+4.00\,\text{DC} \times 50}$$

d
$$\frac{-1.75\,\text{DS}}{-1.00\,\text{DC} \times 140/+4.00\,\text{DC} \times 50}$$

e
$$\frac{-1.75\,\text{DS}}{-1.00\,\text{DC} \times 140/-4.00\,\text{DC} \times 50}$$

Geometric optics

Answers

1 a **True.** The second law of reflection states that the angle of incidence equals the angle of reflection.
  b **False.** The image is laterally inverted and virtual.
  c **False.** A concave mirror forms a virtual image only when the object is placed inside the principal focus. Outside the principal focus, a real image is formed.
  d **True.** A convex mirror forms a virtual, erect, and diminished image.
  e **True.** Convex mirrors are therefore used as car mirrors.

2 a **False.** Sin i/Sin r = the refractive index of the medium.
  b **True.** When light passes through a more dense medium its velocity reduces and the wave is deviated towards the normal.
  c **True.** Refractive index = n = Velocity of light in vacuum/Velocity of light in medium.
  d **True.** When the angle of incidence equals the critical angle the refracted ray runs parallel to the interface.
  e **True.** When the incident ray strikes the interface more obliquely than the critical angle total internal reflection occurs, e.g. angle of the anterior chamber and peripheral retina.

3 a **True.**
  b **False.** A crown glass has a refractive index of 1.52 while flint glass has an index of 1.6.
  c **True.**
  d **False.** The teaching mirror relies on a small proportion of light which is reflected at its anterior surface.
  e **False.** Frequency is invariant.

4 a **True.** The second law of reflection states that the angle of incidence equals the angle of reflection.

b **False.** Snell's law of refraction states that the angles of incidence and refraction are related to the refractive index of the refracting medium and that the incident, reflected, and normal rays all lie in the same plane.

c **False.** Reflection by a plane mirror gives an *erect*, virtual, and laterally inverted image which is equidistant to the mirror as the object.

d **True.**

e **True.**

5 a **True.** An irregular reflecting surface scatters light in many directions. This is diffuse reflection.

b **True.**

c **True.** It has positive, or converging power.

d **True.** Whereas virtual images cannot be captured on a screen.

e **False.** Plane mirrors add no vergence to light, but simply reverse its direction.

6 Make sure you are familiar with the simple ray diagrams required to answer these questions.

a **True.**

b **False.** The image is inverted.

c **True.**

d **True.**

e **False.** The image is magnified.

7 a **False.** The image is virtual.

b **True.**

c **False.** The image is diminished.

d **True.**

e **False.** The image is located at a variable distance from the mirror, depending on the distance of the object.

8 a **True.** Prisms are excellent reflectors and rely on the principle of total internal reflection.

  b **True.**

  c **False.** Owing to total internal reflection. Most of the loss is due to absorption.

  d **True.**

  e **False.** The largest mirror (oblong) in the Goldmann-triple mirror lens gives a view of the equatorial retina, while the gonioscopic mirror (dome-shaped) is used to visualise the angle and pars plana in the dilated eye. The peripheral mirror (square-shaped) gives a view of the retinal periphery between the equator and ora serrata whereas the central part provides a 30 degree view of the posterior pole.

9 a **True.**

  b **False.** The image is inverted.

  c **True.**

  d **False.** The image lies between C and the principal focus.

  e **True.**

10 a **False.** Lens thickness may be ignored in thin lenses.

  b **True.**

  c **True.**

  d **False.** The *first* principal focus is the point of origin of rays which become parallel to the principal axis after refraction by a lens. The *second* principal focus is the point to which parallel light rays converge following refraction by a spherical lens.

  e **False.** Vergence power is the reciprocal of the second focal length in metres.

11 a **True.** Prismatic effect increases towards the periphery of a lens as the refracting angle increases towards the lens edges and may cause ring scotomas and jack-in-the-box effects which are especially troublesome with high refractive errors.

  b **True.**

  c **True.** Prismatic effect is calculated using the formula $P = DF$ where P is the prism power in dioptres, D is the decentration in *centimetres* and F is the lens power in dioptres (Prentice rule).

  d **False.** The prismatic effect of the downward decentration of a $+12$ dioptre lens by 3 mm is 3.6 D base *down*.

  e **False.** Upward decentration of a -6 dioptre lens by 5 mm causes a 3 D base *down* prismatic effect.

12 a **True.** This is a working definition of a thin lens. In practice, we would also need to know the required accuracy of any calculation – for a high degree of accuracy, thin lens approximations cannot be used.

b **False.** If a low power lens has large physical thickness, then it cannot be considered *thin*.

c **False.**

d **False.** We cannot consider a lens of 3 mm thickness as *thin* unless we also know its focal length, and the object and image distances.

e **False.** Refractive index does not determine whether a lens can be considered *thin*; a lens of *low* refractive index will tend to be physically thicker for a particular focal length (i.e., not thin) and a lens of high refractive index will have a shorter focal length for a particular thickness (i.e., not thin).

13 a **True.** The powers of thin lenses in contact can be added together. The power of this combination would be $(+2) + (-1) = +1$ DS: the focal length is the inverse of the power in dioptres, and is therefore 1 metre.

b **False.** A Galilean telescope is made by combining a concave and a convex lens so that the first focal point of the concave lens is coincident with the second focal point of the convex lens. This requires the power of the concave lens to be higher than that of the convex lens. Therefore, a Galilean telescope cannot be made from these two lenses.

c **False.** A real image is formed 0.50 m from the lens.

d **True.**

e **False.** An image (virtual) is formed -0.33 m from the lens.

14 a **True.** An angle of deviation (D) is half the refracting or apical angle (A) of a prism, according to the formula $D = (n - 1)A$, where n is the refractive index.

b **False.** Light refracted by a prism is deviated towards the base of a prism but the image is deviated towards the apex and is virtual and erect.

c **False.** The position of minimum deviation is such that the angle of incidence equals the angle of emergence and refraction is symmetrical.

d **True.** In the Prentice position, one surface of the prism is perpendicular to the incident ray so that all refraction occurs at the other surface.

e **True.**

15 a **False.** The displacement produced by a "centrad" is measured along an arc *1 metre* from the prism.

  b **False.** The "centrad" produces a slightly greater angle of deviation.

  c **True.** When a prism is placed before a seeing eye, the eye will move to regain fixation.

  d **True.**

  e **False.** High powered cylinders.

16 a **False.** The Rodenstock panfundoscope consists of a high power convex lens. No prism is incorporated in this contact lens.

  b **True.**

  c **True.**

  d **True.**

  e **False.**

17 a **False.** The combined power of two prisms stacked on top of one another is not equal to the sum of their individual powers due to the fact that light incident on the second prism will already have been refracted by the first prism and hence will not be at the correct angle of incidence.

  b **False.** A prism of power 6 D deviates light through 3.43 degrees and has an apical angle of 6.86 degrees assuming that its refractive index is 1.5.

  c **False.** Power is approximately 25Δ in this case.

  d **False.** A 1Δ prism produces a linear apparent displacement of *1 cm* of an object at *1 m*.

  e **True.**

18 a **True.** Fresnel prisms are plastic prisms stuck onto the back surface of ordinary spectacle lenses.

  b **True.** Visual acuity may suffer due to scattering of light. Chromatic aberration also affects vision, especially in the high prism powers.

  c **True.**

  d **False.** They are designed for temporary use only.

  e **False.** They consist of a sheet of tiny parallel prisms of *identical* power.

19 a **True.**
  b **True.** When using prisms therapeutically, the prismatic correction is usually shared between the two eyes. To correct a horizontal deviation the orientation of the prisms is identical for both eyes. To correct a vertical deviation the prism arrangement must be opposite in both eyes.
  c **False.** Hence to correct a 10 D right hypotropia requires a 5Δ base up prism for the right eye and a 5Δ base down prism for the left eye.
  d **True.** The image is displaced towards the apex of the prism. Thus the apex of the prism should be placed towards the direction of deviation of an eye.
  e **True.**

20 a **False.** Porro prisms deviate light through 180 degrees and vertically invert but do not laterally invert the image. They are used to shorten instruments, e.g. the slit lamp microscope, but are not right-angled.
  b **False.** Dove prisms vertically invert but do not laterally invert the image.
  c **True.**
  d **True.**
  e **True.** The Goldmann tonometer head contains 2 *base out* prisms.

21 a **False.** Light entering a more dense medium is deviated towards the normal.
  b **True.**
  c **False.** Snell's law states that the incident ray, the refracted ray, and the normal are in the same plane and that $n = \mathrm{Sin}\, i / \mathrm{Sin}\, r$.
  d **False.**
  e **True.** The direction of light passing through a glass plane obliquely is unchanged, but the light is laterally displaced.

22 a **True.**
  b **True.**
  c **False.** The vergence power of a curved interface is $(n_1 - n_2)/r$.
  d **False.** The surface power is positive for a converging surface and negative for a diverging surface.
  e **True.**

23 a True.
    b False. They are the meridians of maximum *and* minimum curvature.
    c True.
    d True.
    e False. Both the direction of the axis and the strength of the cylinder may be defined.

24 a True.
    b False. The handle is at 45 degrees to the axes.
    c True.
    d True. While a 1.0 DC cross cylinder is used for a patient with poor vision.
    e True.

25 a False. The phenomenon of apparent depth occurs when objects are viewed while immersed in a medium of greater optic density than that being viewed from. Rays emerging from the object towards the observer are refracted at the interface between the two media and create a virtual image which appears less deep than the object is. This is important in intra-ocular surgery.
    b False.
    c True.
    d True.
    e True. Total internal reflection is utilised in fibreoptic cables and in the eye; it prevents visualisation of certain structures such as the peripheral retina and the trabecular meshwork.

26 a True. Gonioscope contact lenses are made of a material with a higher refractive index than the eye and the use of a coupling fluid neutralises the cornea:air refracting interface. This overcomes total internal reflection, allowing visualisation of the angle and peripheral retina.
    b True.
    c False. The Zeiss goniolens is applied directly to the cornea without a coupling fluid because it is flatter than the cornea.
    d True. For this reason the lens must be used with a coupling fluid.
    e False. The Koeppe is a direct goniolens and its particular benefit is that it allows a synchronous comparison of the two angles.

27 a **True.**
    b **False.** Short wavelength light (e.g. blue) is deviated more than long wavelength light.
    c **True.**
    d **True.**
    e **True.**

28 a **False.** Chromatic aberration accounts for approximately 1.5–2.0 D of aberration in the eye.
    b **False.** The dispersive power of a material is independent of its refractive index.
    c **True.**
    d **True.**
    e **False.** The duochrome test depends on the position of the image with respect to the retina. A colour blind patient should be asked whether the upper or lower rank of letters appears clearer.

29 a **True.** "Stops" eliminate rays passing through the peripheral zone of a spherical lens and thereby reduce spherical aberration.
    b **False.** In a spherical lens the prismatic effect is least in the paraxial zone and rays passing through this region are refracted less than those passing through the peripheral zone.
    c **True.** With a dilated pupil, a significant amount of light passes through the periphery of the lens and therefore contributes to spherical aberration.
    d **True.**
    e **False.** Spherical aberration is increased with a biconvex lens.

30 a **True.**
    b **True.** The astigmatic image formed in the human eye falls on the peripheral retina where there are few cones as compared to the macula. Owing to the poor resolution of the image in the peripheral retina the effect of oblique astigmatism in the human eye is thereby reduced.
    c **False.** Coma is a variant of spherical aberration.
    d **True.**
    e **True.**

31 a **False.** Achromatic lenses correct chromatic aberration. Aplanatic lenses correct spherical aberration.

   b **True.** Doublets consist of a principal lens and a weaker lens of different refractive index and opposite power.

   c **True.** The weaker lens being of opposite power reduces the power at the periphery of the principal lens and thereby reduces spherical aberration. The difference in refractive indices of the two lenses reduces chromatic aberration, as it can be designed that they produce opposite amounts of dispersion.

   d **True.**

   e **True.**

32 a **False.** A pin-cushion effect is typical of a high power convex lens (e.g., for the correction of aphakia).

   b **False.** The jack-in-the-box phenomenon is explained by the "ring scotoma" produced by the prismatic effect at the edge of a lens.

   c **True.**

   d **True.** The curvature of a field depends upon the refractive index of the lens material and the curvature of the lens surface.

   e **True.**

33 a **True.** It measures the surface curvature of lenses to give their power.

   b **True.**

   c **False.** It is calibrated for crown glass.

   d **False.** This is the focimeter.

   e **False.**

34 d is correct.

35 b is correct.

36 d is correct.

37 b is correct.

   a is the toric transposition to a -6.00 base curve.

38 d is correct.
   c is correct for a sphere curve of -6.
   e is correct for a sphere curve of $+6$.

39 d is correct.

40 c is correct.

41 a is correct.

42 c is correct.

43 c is correct.

44 c is correct.

45 a is correct.

46 d is correct.

47 c is correct.

48 a is correct.

Clinical optics

Questions

1 The resolution of the visual system:

   a Is related to visual acuity.
   b Is maximised by pupil diameters below 1 mm.
   c Can alter greatly depending on the level of ambient illumination.
   d Is related to contrast sensitivity.
   e Is reduced by a lens opacity which affects the visual axis.

2 The Stiles–Crawford (S–C) effect:

   a Explains the Purkinje shift.
   b Reduces the effect of the optical aberrations of the eye on vision.
   c Is less evident in the case of an amblyopic eye.
   d Results because the photoreceptors are roughly aligned towards the second focal point of the eye.
   e Results in a reduction in sensitivity to rays of light which enter the eye parallel to the visual axis, but through the periphery of the pupil.

3 In Gullstrand's schematic eye:

   a There are two principal points in the anterior chamber.
   b There are two nodal points at the posterior pole of the lens.
   c The refractive power is $+58.6$ D.
   d Nodal points coincide with the principal points.
   e The first principal point is 3 mm behind the anterior corneal surface.

4 The reduced eye has:

a A refractive power of $+58.6\,D$.
b A single nodal point at the posterior pole of the lens.
c A single principal point in the anterior chamber.
d The second focal point falls on the retina in emmetropia.
e The first focal point is 17.5 mm in front of the cornea.

5 Visual acuity

The following are true:

a The standard of normal visual acuity is 5 minutes of arc.
b Each letter on the Snellen chart subtends an angle of 5 minutes at the distance specified for it.
c Visual acuity is expressed as a ratio where the numerator is the distance in metres at which the test type is read.
d Visual acuity of 6/24 on the Snellen's chart is exactly equivalent to 3/12.
e The illumination of the test types is an important factor.

6 Visual acuity in a patient who is unable to recognise letters is assessed by:

a Snellen's chart.
b Log Mar chart.
c Landolt's broken ring test.
d E test.
e Vistech chart.

7 Near visual acuity is tested using:

a Reduced Snellen's.
b Jaeger's test type.
c Cambridge chart.
d Worth's four-dot test.
e Frisby test.

8 Visual acuity in infants aged one year may be roughly estimated with:

    a Sheridan Gardiner test type.
    b Kay pictures.
    c Keeler acuity cards.
    d Teller cards.
    e Cardiff acuity tests.

9 Accommodation:

    a In the non-presbyope, fluctuates continuously by about 0.25 DS.
    b May be slower and less accurate under monochromatic illumination.
    c For a moderate hypermetrope, is subjectively greater in amplitude in contact lens than in spectacle correction.
    d Only decreases measurably with age after the age of 25 years.
    e Cannot occur without a change in pupil size.

10 The AC/A ratio:

    a Can be measured using fixation disparities.
    b When measured by the gradient method, using cover tests at 1/3 m, is normally of the order of 10:1 (prism dioptres/DS).
    c Does not increase with pupil size, when measured subjectively.
    d Cannot be measured at 6 m.
    e Response AC/A ratios are measured clinically.

11 Regarding refracting a patient complaining of blurred vision:

    a Accommodative excess may result in a convergent squint.
    b Accommodative excess should be treated with bifocals if possible.
    c Pinhole acuity should be better than unaided vision in cases with refractive error.
    d Irregular astigmatism can only be detected by keratometry or corneal topography.
    e If the patient is a contact lens wearer, lenses should be removed for at least a week before refraction for spectacles can be considered.

12 Regarding refractive surgery:

a Radial keratotomy increases myopia by flattening the cornea.
b Radial keratotomy is indicated in patients with at least 8 dioptres of myopia.
c Epikeratophakia may be used to treat keratoconus.
d Epikeratophakia is only useful for stable myopia of between 2 and 8 dioptres.
e Contraindications of epikeratophakia include lagophthalmos.

13 Regarding intra-ocular lenses (IOLs):

a The power of an IOL in air is of the order of 80 D.
b The power of an IOL in the eye is of the order of 20 D.
c The reduced power of an IOL in the eye compared with in air is due to the fact that the refractive index of air is greater than that of aqueous.
d IOL power may be approximated with a ruler.
e IOL power is the reciprocal of its focal length.

14 For a particular patient, A-scan biometry and keratometry are performed before cataract surgery, and an IOL is selected with the intention of producing emmetropia:

a If the axial length was under-estimated by 1 mm, the patient would be about 1 D myopic following surgery.
b If the intra-ocular lens was placed posterior to the desired position (deep anterior chamber following surgery) the patient would be hypermetropic following surgery.
c If an appropriate anterior chamber lens was used in the right eye, and an appropriate posterior chamber lens in the left eye, the patient may experience images in the left eye as being slightly larger.
d A change of 1 mm in axial length would have less effect on refraction than a change of 1 mm in central corneal radius.
e Astigmatism after surgery could be due to the A-scan being performed significantly off-axis.

15 Regarding IOL calculation:

   a The SRK(T) formula is not suitable for eyes with an axial length of 25 mm or longer.
   b The SRK formula is used to calculate IOL power.
   c The SRK formula has A, B, and C constants which are usually 118.5, 0.9, and 2.5 respectively.
   d The D constant, which is always 1.25, may be used to calculate refractive states other than emmetropia.
   e The SRK formula is accurate for a very small range of axial lengths.

16 The following are true:

   a An IOL overcomes the aneisokonia produced with spectacle correction of aphakia.
   b The relative spectacle magnification with an IOL is greater than with a contact lens used to correct the same refractive error.
   c An IOL is an equi-convex lens with spherical surfaces.
   d A high myope may be rendered emmetropic by aphakic cataract extraction.
   e A +12 dioptre contact lens may be suitable for an aphake.

17 Problems associated with spectacle correction of aphakia include:

   a Discomfort.
   b Misjudgement of distances due to aneisokonia.
   c Reduced performance on visual acuity tests.
   d A ring scotoma.
   e A small field of vision.

18 Correction of unilateral aphakia:

   a With spectacles causes aneisokonia.
   b With spectacles gives a relative spectacle magnification of 1.1.
   c With contact lenses gives a relative spectacle magnification of 1.3.
   d With an IOL gives a relative spectacle magnification of 1.1.
   e Is best with an iseikonic lens.

19 Best form lenses:

 a Reduce spherical aberration.
 b Include meniscus and periscopic lenses.
 c Reduce chromatic aberrations.
 d The base curve of a positive lens is positive.
 e The concave surface is always placed next to the eye.

20 Spectacle intolerance is commonly associated with:

 a Anisometropia.
 b A difference of 40 degrees between the cylindrical axes of the two eyes.
 c High refractive errors.
 d Amblyopia.
 e Bifocals.

21 Bifocals

The following are true:

 a Fused bifocals incorporate a near segment of crown glass.
 b Image jump may be overcome by ensuring the optical centres of the near and distance portions lie at or near their junction.
 c Image displacement is explained by prismatic effect.
 d Bifocals are unsuitable in high oblique astigmatism.
 e Image jump is reduced in flat-topped bifocals.

22 Regarding progressive addition lenses:

 a Peripheral field of vision is distorted by oblique astigmatism.
 b Oblique astigmatism is reduced with soft multifocal lenses.
 c A narrow corridor between near and distance portions is used for intermediate viewing.
 d They are well accepted by most patients.
 e They eliminate image jump.

43

23 Spectacle lenses

The following are true:

a PMMA is susceptible to scratching.
b The effective power of a positive lens increases as it is moved away from the eye.
c A stronger positive lens is required at the cornea of the eye than at the spectacle plane.
d Orthoscopic lenses relieve an equal amount of convergence and accommodation.
e In aphakia, peripheral vision is improved by rotoid lenses.

24 A bilaterally aphakic patient can see 6/5 in each eye with contact lenses of power $+18$ DS

The following are true:

a In place of contact lenses, the patient would require spectacles with lenses of a higher power than $+18$ DS for distance vision.
b If the right contact lens could not be worn, the patient would be best corrected with a contact lens of power $+18$ DS in the left eye, and a spectacle lens of between $+8$ DS and $+18$ DS in front of the right eye.
c The patient's visual field would appear larger in contact lenses than spectacles.
d The patient's visual acuity would be better than 6/5 in spectacles.
e The patient will experience a magnification effect on switching to spectacles.

25 An emmetropic patient is fitted with a concave contact lens and a $+10$ DS spectacle lens at a back vertex distance of 20 mm. The contact lens power is chosen in order to allow clear vision at 6 m

The following are true:

a In order to see clearly at 6 m, the contact lens power will be -12.5 DS.
b A contact lens of power -12.50 DS is only available as a soft lens.
c This device will partially stabilise the retinal image in the presence of eye movements.
d This device will produce magnification of the order of 10%.
e This device will only allow clear vision at 33 cm if the patient reduces the back vertex distance of the spectacle lens.

26 Contact lenses

The following are true:

a Astigmatism in excess of 5 dioptres cannot be adequately corrected using contact lenses.
b Hard contact lenses contain about 5% water at room temperature.
c A tear pump effect is only necessary with hard lenses.
d Although soft lenses can be reground, the same is not true of hard or gas permeable materials.
e For rigid contact lenses, a change of 0.05 mm in the back central optic radius can be expected to result in a change of approximately 0.25 D of refractive correction.

27 In the case of soft contact lenses:

a If vision is clearer immediately after blinking, then the contact lens is probably too steep.
b A thick lens is best fitted tight.
c Prisms cannot be incorporated into the prescription.
d Soft contact lenses are unsuitable for children.
e A reduction in atmospheric humidity (such as in a pressurised aeroplane cabin) may lead to a tightening of lens fit.

28 The ideal contact lens material would:

a Have a high Dk value.
b Have a low wetting angle.
c Have a refractive index below 1.4.
d Have a low density.
e Have high dispersive power.

29 The following are advantages of the optics of contact lenses over spectacles:

a The optical centres of contact lenses remain near the visual axis.
b The field of view is increased for hypermetropic patients.
c Less accommodation is required for myopic patients.
d Less vergence is required for hypermetropic patients.
e Because they sit closer to the nodal point of the eye, magnification effects are reduced.

30 The following patients are often able to be better corrected using spectacles than contact lenses:

a A 30-year-old with moderate keratoconus.
b A 30-year-old deep sea diver.
c A patient with aphakia in one eye, myopia in the other, and equal visual acuity in each eye. ᵛ
d A 4-year-old child with divergence excess.
e A patient with Down's syndrome.

31 Contact lenses

The following are true:

a The base curve of a contact lens is the curvature of the central portion of the back surface of the lens.
b A high plus contact lens has a central thin portion.
c A ballasted lens has a heavier base which lies inferiorly *in situ* on the cornea.
d Hard lenses abolish lenticular astigmatism.
e In scleral lenses the haptic is the corneal portion.

32 Regarding oxygen permeability:

a Oxygen flux is proportional to the Dk value.
b Oxygen flux is inversely proportional to the lens thickness and partial pressure drop across the lens.
c PMMA and HEMA are low flux materials.
d High water content hydrogel lenses are high flux materials.
e Equivalent oxygen performance is a measure of O_2 permeability *in vivo*.

33 Cornea

The following are true:

a The corneal apex is the area of maximum curvature of the cornea and is about 4 mm diameter.
b Spectacle blur refers to the visual blurring on removal of a contact lens and may be due to altered corneal astigmatism.
c Contact lenses induce a predominant anaerobic metabolism in the corneal epithelium.
d Contact lenses cause an adaptive reduction in corneal sensation.
e Soft lenses always abolish astigmatism.

34 Rigid contact lenses

The following are true:

a PMMA lenses are usually small corneal lenses.
b While wearing PMMA lenses, 90% of the oxygen required by the cornea is derived from transfer through the lens.
c Silicone rubber is an example of a gas permeable lens material.
d Gas permeable lenses can correct several dioptres of astigmatism while maintaining corneal deturgesence.
e Gas permeable lenses may be bifocal.

35 Regarding contact lens fitting:

a Contact lenses are fitted using minus cylinders.
b BVD is not required to calculate contact lens power from spectacle lens power.
c Spherical soft contact lenses cannot be used where corneal astigmatism is greater than 1 D.
d The most important factor in determining if a patient is suitable for soft contact lenses is the presence or absence of significant total astigmatism.
e Contact lenses are contraindicated in glaucoma.

47

36 Regarding contact lens fitting:

    a The smaller the diameter, the tighter a contact lens will be.

    b 8–9 mm is the recommended diameter for gas permeable lenses.

    c 8–9 mm is the recommended diameter for PMMA lenses.

    d Keratoconus produces a central bright green patch and peripheral dark pooling in contact lens fluorescein pattern evaluation.

    e Lenticular astigmatism is measured by subtracting the corneal astigmatism from the total astigmatism found on refraction.

37 Gas permeable (GP) contact lenses:

    a Are more comfortable than hard lenses.

    b Are associated with a greater incidence of complications than soft lenses.

    c Are more durable than soft lenses.

    d May have an almost flat anterior surface in high myopes.

    e Often require fenestrations.

38 Regarding soft contact lenses:

    a They are easily damaged.

    b Fluctuating vision can be an indication of how the lens is fitting.

    c Spherical lenses may cause reduced visual acuity in patients with high astigmatism.

    d Increasing the base curve radius increases the lens tightness.

    e Increasing the lens diameter increases the lens movement.

39 The following are signs of a loose fitting soft contact lens:

    a Mucous threads in the tear film.

    b Blanching of the conjunctival blood vessels.

    c 2 mm of lag on upgaze and versions.

    d 3 and 9 o'clock conjunctival staining.

    e If pushed off the cornea, the lens re-centres on the cornea within 1 second.

40 Extended wear contact lenses:

    a Have a small diameter to optimise stability and vision.
    b Minimise hand contamination.
    c Increase chemical toxicity.
    d May be problematic for patients with dry eyes.
    e Usually need to be changed weekly.

41 The following options are possible for a contact lens wearing presbyopic patient, who wishes to see clearly for distance and near tasks:

    a Monovision contact lenses.
    b Progressive addition contact lenses.
    c Solid bifocal contact lenses.
    d Diffractive bifocal contact lenses.
    e Pinhole contact lenses.

42 The following patients might be expected to report that their vision is better using contact lenses, compared to spectacles:

    a A patient with 4 dioptres of oblique astigmatism in each eye.
    b A patient with early keratoconus in both eyes.
    c A patient with a large face turn associated with congenital nystagmus, and 4 dioptres of myopia in each eye.
    d A patient with 10 dioptres of myopia in both eyes.
    e A patient with 1 dioptre of hypermetropia.

43 Contact lenses

The following are true:

    a In the case of a high myope, the required contact lens power will exceed the power of the spectacles lens.
    b Corneal lenses are commonly fenestrated to improve oxygen flux.
    c The retinal image is more magnified using contact lenses than spectacles in the case of a hypermetropic patient.
    d If fitted with an RGP lens, a toric design will be required for a patient with corneal astigmatism equal to spectacle astigmatism.
    e If fitted with an ultra-thin soft lens, a toric design will be required for a patient with corneal astigmatism, but no spectacle astigmatism.

44 Contact lens care

The following are true:

a Deposits may cause giant papillary conjunctivitis.
b A rinsing solution is required *before* cleaning with surfactants.
c Deposits may reduce oxygen transmission.
d Thiomersal is a preservative which may cause allergy.
e Most preparations are active against acanthamoeba.

45 Low visual aids

The following are true:

a Low visual aids are designed for near vision only.
b Low visual aids act by increasing the angle subtended at the eye by the object.
c A simple magnifier is a powerful concave lens.
d The object is placed at the nodal point of a hand-held magnifier.
e A simple magnifier forms a virtual image.

46 Simple magnifiers

The following are true:

a As the object moves closer to the principal focus, the image becomes larger.
b A paperweight or dome magnifier is a plano-convex lens.
c A convex cylindrical lens with the axis of the cylinder horizontal is used as a magnifier.
d A high powered magnifier is held farther from the page than a low powered lens.
e Effective magnification of a lens is approximately 4 times its dioptric power.

47 Regarding magnifiers:

   a Fresnel lenses are used as magnifiers.
   b The head band loupe incorporates base out prisms.
   c The object is at the anterior focal point of the spectacle borne visual aid.
   d Marked spherical aberration is a disadvantage of Fresnel lenses, compared to a solid lens.
   e The field of vision depends on the aperture of the lens.

48 Regarding the optical characteristics of a simple magnifier:

   a The field of view decreases as magnification is increased.
   b Depth of focus increases with increasing magnification.
   c Greater magnification requires less illumination.
   d When the object is at the principal focus the image is erect.
   e When the object is outside the principal focus the image is inverted and diminished.

49 The Galilean telescope:

   a Works on the same principle as the astronomical telescope.
   b Has two convex lenses separated by the sum of their focal lengths.
   c Forms an erect, magnified, real image.
   d Can be adapted for near and distance vision.
   e Has a field of view relatively free from astigmatism.

50 An astronomical telescope:

   a Has two convex lenses.
   b Has lenses separated by the sum of their focal lengths.
   c Forms an inverted real image.
   d Can be used for near vision with the addition of a convex lens held near to the objective.
   e Views an object outside the principal focus of the objective.

51 Regarding magnification:

    a Magnification of a telescope is the ratio of the dioptric power of the objective to that of the eye piece.

    b A concave contact lens in combination with a convex spectacle lens acts as a telescopic system.

    c Doublets of up to 80 dioptres power may be used as spectacle magnifiers.

    d High power spectacle magnifiers incorporate base out prisms.

    e A Galilean telescope inverted gives the subject an increased field of view.

52 Low vision

The following are true:

    a Patients with low vision may benefit from reversed contrast.

    b CCTV offers magnification of up to 40 times.

    c A stenopaeic (Knapp's) glass is more effective than a stenopaeic hole.

    d Distance visual acuity in the partially sighted is tested using the Lovie–Bailey chart.

    e A horizontal stenopaeic slit protects against UV radiation.

53 Fresnel lenses:

    a May be used as low vision aids.

    b Were used in lighthouses.

    c May cause a reduction in visual acuity.

    d Reduce aberrations.

    e Are heavier than ordinary spherical lenses.

54 An emmetropic patient has an amplitude of accommodation of 1.50 D measured using the RAF rule. The patient works for 6 hours each day at a VDU screen at a distance of 50 cm, and views reading material at a distance of 33 cm

The following are true:

a This patient is likely to be about 45 years old in light of the accommodative amplitude.

b For viewing the VDU screen, no lens will be required, in theory.

c For viewing reading material, a reading addition of +2.25 DS is likely to be required.

d Bifocals of power +1.25 DS with an addition of +1 DS would theoretically suit this patient if she wished to have only one pair of glasses.

e Trifocal lenses would be unsuitable for this patient.

Clinical optics

Answers

1 a **True.**
   b **False.** Very small pupil diameters result in a loss of resolution due to diffractive effects.
   c **True.** At scotopic levels, when only rods are functioning, visual acuity is much reduced.
   d **True.** This effect is most noticeable at high spatial frequencies, when contrast sensitivity equates to visual acuity.
   e **True.**

2 a **False.** The Purkinje shift is due to the different spectral sensitivities of rods and cones, and results in a shift in the peak of the spectral sensitivity curve on going from photopic to scotopic levels of illumination.
   b **True.** Because the S–C effect reduces sensitivity to blurred images.
   c **True.** Anatomical studies have shown that in the retinae of amblyopes, the S–C effect is absent or reduced.
   d **False.** The photoreceptors point towards the nodal point of the eye.
   e **True.**

3 a **True.** The two principal points lie 1.35 mm and 1.60 mm behind the anterior corneal surface.
   b **False.** The two nodal points straddle the posterior pole of the lens.
   c **True.**
   d **False.** As the media on either side of the refracting system of the eye are different, i.e. air ($n = 1$) and vitreous ($n = 1.336$), the nodal and principal points do not coincide.
   e **False.**

4 a **True.**
  b **True.** The nodal point lies 7.08 mm behind the anterior corneal surface, i.e. on the posterior pole of the lens.
  c **True.** The principal point is 1.35 mm behind the anterior corneal surface.
  d **True.** The second focal point is 24.13 mm behind the anterior corneal surface and this lies on the retina in emmetropia.
  e **False.** It lies 15.7 mm in front of the cornea.

5 a **False.** The standard limit of visual acuity is 1 minute of arc.
  b **True.** Each "limb" of the letter on the Snellen chart subtends an angle of 1 minute of arc at the specified distance. The whole letter subtends an angle of 5 minutes of arc.
  c **True.**
  d **False.** 6/24 on a Lovie–Bailey chart, however, is equivalent to 3/12, as it addresses the problem of spacing between letters with respect to their size.
  e **True.** When the illumination falls below 2 lumens/sq foot, the efficiency of the normal eye falls very rapidly. The ideal standard is about 50 lumens/sq foot.

6 a **False.** Snellen's chart employs letters as does the Log Mar chart and both are therefore of little value for an illiterate subject.
  b **False.**
  c **True.** The patient is instructed to indicate the orientation of each broken ring.
  d **True.** A chart with the letter "E" of varying sizes and facing in varying directions is displayed. The patient is given a wooden "E" which he holds in the same direction as the test type.
  e **False.** Vistech charts are used to assess contrast sensitivity.

7 a **True.** The standard Snellen types are reduced to approximately 1/17 of their normal size and the chart is held at a distance of approximately 35 cm.
  b **True.** Jaeger's test type uses varying sizes of ordinary printer's fonts.
  c **False.** The Cambridge chart is used to test contrast sensitivity.
  d **False.** This is a suppression test.
  e **False.** The Frisby test is a test of stereopsis.

8 a **False.** Sheridan Gardiner test requires the recognition of letters and cannot be used in young infants.

  b **False.** Kay pictures test requires the child to recognise and match pictures. This can usually be carried out by the age of 2.

  c **True.** Keeler acuity cards use gratings of varying spatial frequency. This is a preferential looking test and is suitable in infants under 12 months.

  d **True.** The Teller card is very similar to the Keeler card and can be employed in the same age group. The former however takes less time to perform.

  e **True.** This uses the preferential looking principle but has pictures.

9 a **True.**

  b **True.** This is thought to be because under monochromatic illumination the accommodation system cannot use the transverse chromatic aberration of the eye to give information on the direction of dioptric blur – in other words, initially, the accommodation system does not know whether to relax or to accommodate.

  c **True.** This is due to the increased effectivity of spectacles compared to contact lenses.

  d **False.** Measurable (rather than clinically relevant) reductions in amplitude can be detected as early as 8–10 years of age.

  e **False.** Studies have shown that accommodation can occur (in normal subjects) without a corresponding pupillary constriction.

10 a **True.**

  b **False.** A normal AC/A ratio will usually be below 4:1 under these circumstances.

  c **False.** As pupil size increases, more accommodation is normally required, and the AC/A ratio therefore appears to increase.

  d **False.** Would be required for a set distance.

  e **False.** Response AC/A ratios are measured by using an objective measure of accommodative response. Stimulus AC/A ratios are measured clinically.

11 a True.
  b False. The treatment of choice would be orthoptic exercises, or single vision spectacles to correct any distance hypermetropia.
  c True. This is because the use of the pinhole reduces blur.
  d False. The retinoscope also detects irregular astigmatism.
  e False. Soft contact lens wearers can almost always be accurately refracted immediately after removal of lenses. Corneal effects are more common with PMMA lens wearers, but even many of these undergo only a small change on removal of lenses. In addition to these considerations, if the patient is intending to use the spectacles immediately after contact lens use, then this would be the optimum time to refract them!

12 a False. Radial keratotomy *decreases* myopia by flattening the cornea.
  b False. These patients are unsuitable because their final refractive correction is unpredictable.
  c True. It may also be useful for young children with monocular aphakia. Astigmatism and other problems limit its effectiveness.
  d False. These are the criteria for radial keratotomy. Epikeratophakia can correct any degree of myopia and hypermetropia up to 27 dioptres (aphakia).
  e True. Other contraindications include dry eyes and patients with less than 4 dioptres of myopia, in which radial keratotomy is preferable.

13 a True. The power of a standard IOL is much greater than in the eye due to the greater discrepancy in the air:lens refractive index ratios compared with the aqueous:lens refractive index ratios.
  b True.
  c False. The refractive index of air is less than that of aqueous, i.e. the ratio $n_{air}:n_{lens}$ is less than the ratio $n_{aqueous}:n_{lens}$.
  d True. If parallel light, for example from a light bulb, is brought to focus by an IOL in air, the distance between the lens and its focal point is its focal length and the inverse of this is the lens power.
  e True.

14 a False. Such an error would result in closer to 3 D of myopia.
 b True.
 c False. An anterior chamber lens produces slight magnification of the retinal image, compared to a posterior chamber lens.
 d True. The effect of a corneal radius change of 1 mm would be of the order of 6 D (depending on the actual radius). Axial length errors are more likely to occur than keratometry errors, and 1 mm error gives an error of approximately 3 D.
 e False.

15 a False.
 b True.
 c False. The SRK formula is widely used to calculate IOL power. Its formula states that

$$P = A - B(AL) - C(K)$$

where P = the IOL power in dioptres
A = the constant associated with IOL model, usually 118.5
B = the multiplication constant for axial length, usually 2.5
AL = the axial length in mm
C = the multiplication constant for the average keratometry reading, approx. 0.9
K = the average keratometry reading

 d False. The D constant is 1.25 if the IOL power for emmetropia is 14 dioptres and 1.0 if less than 14 dioptres.
 e False. The SRK formula is accurate for a large range of axial lengths.

16 a True. Use of an IOL in aphakia overcomes the aneisokonia produced with spectacle correction of aphakia as the IOL causes minimal magnification effects because it is situated near the natural position of the crystalline lens.
 b False. The relative spectacle magnification with an IOL is 1.0 while with a contact lens it is 1.1.
 c False. An IOL is a bi-convex lens, with aspherical surfaces. The anterior surface is normally flatter than the posterior surface.
 d True. Aphakia is equivalent to high hypermetropia, therefore a high myope may be rendered emmetropic by aphakic cataract extraction.
 e True. Contact lens powers in aphakia are normally in the range of +10–18 dioptres. In young babies, a contact lens of the order of +40 dioptres may be required.

17 a True. Aphakic spectacles are heavy and tend to slip.

  b True. Uneven image magnification causes aneisokonia and misjudging of distances, which can be dangerous.

  c False. Image magnification may lead to an *enhanced* performance on visual acuity tests.

  d True. The ring scotoma, or jack-in-the-box effect, are caused by the prismatic effect of the lens.

  e True. Magnification, and the distortion in the peripheral field.

18 a True. Correction of unilateral aphakia with spectacles gives a relative spectacle magnification of 1.33 in the aphakic eye causing aneisokonia and diplopia.

  b False.

  c False. Contact lenses improve the disparity as the relative spectacle magnification is of the order of 1.1.

  d False. Similarly with an IOL the relative spectacle magnification is 1, allowing binocular vision.

  e False. Iseikonic lenses are lenses with no focusing power but which alter the net image size. However, the maximum magnification achievable is 5% and the lenses are expensive and bulky.

19 a True. A best form lens minimises oblique astigmatism and spherical aberration.

  b True. According to its base curve, a best form may be called a "meniscus lens" (base curve of 6 D) or a periscopic lens (base curve of 1.25 D).

  c False. They do not eliminate chromatic aberration.

  d False. A positive best form lens has a negative base curve and vice versa.

  e True.

20 a True. In anisometropia, unequal magnification and unequal prismatic effects give rise to spectacle intolerance.

  b True. Where the axes of the cylinders vary by more than 20 degrees, spectacle intolerance is more common.

  c True. In high myopic or aphakic corrections, the marked prismatic effect at the lens periphery often causes intolerance.

  d False.

  e True. In a bifocal lens, the prismatic effect at the junction of the near and distance segments may initially give rise to some discomfort.

21 a **False.** The distance segment is of crown glass, while the near segment is flint glass of higher refractive index.

   b **True.** When the optical centres lie at or near the junction of the two segments the prismatic effect responsible for image jump is removed.

   c **True.** Image displacement is produced by the prismatic effect seen at parts other than the optical centre of the lens.

   d **True.** Bifocals are unsuitable when there is high oblique astigmatism, marked anisometropia, and muscle imbalance.

   e **True.** Because the optical centre of the bifocal segment is at the junction.

22 a **True.** The lateral parts of progressive addition lenses are subject to considerable aberrations on account of their non-spherical curvature. This leads to a sense of distortion on looking down and to the side, which is exaggerated in the presence of moderate oblique astigmatism. The effective visual field is thereby restricted.

   b **True.** A "soft" multifocal lens is a progressive addition lens with relatively less oblique astigmatism in its lateral parts.

   c **True.**

   d **True.** The restricted effect visual field and distortion on lateral gaze are disconcerting for many users initially, but such drawbacks are outweighed by convenience of this form of lens for most patients.

   e **True.** The gradual accretion of power from the distance to the near portion eliminates image jump.

23 a **True.** PMMA is susceptible to scratching and has a tendency to warp when heated.

   b **True.** When a convex lens is moved away from the eye, its focal length would need to be increased, so that the second focal point of the lens coincides with the far point of the eye. Therefore, a weaker convex lens is now required, i.e. the effective power of the convex lens increases as it is moved away from the eye.

   c **True.**

   d **True.** Orthoscopic lenses are useful in non-presbyopic individuals engaged in very fine work requiring magnification, e.g. watch-repairers, ophthalmic surgery.

   e **True.** A rotoid lens has a steep curve so that the centres of curvature of the two surfaces coincide at the centre of rotation of the eye. This ensures clarity of peripheral vision in aphakia.

24 a **False.**

    b **False.** This would cause intolerable aniseikonia (and/or diplopia) due to the relative magnification effect of the spectacle lens, and the induced prismatic effect when the eyes move into eccentric gaze.

    c **True.** In high hypermetropic spectacle corrections, the visual world is magnified (giving a reduced field of view) and a ring scotoma is produced.

    d **True.** Although unlikely in real life, due to the aberrations inherent in high lens corrections, the magnification produced would give an enhanced acuity in this case.

    e **True.**

25 a **True.** The contact lens power required will be

$$-10/(1 + 0.02(-10)) = -12.50\,\text{DS}$$

    b **False.**

    c **True.**

    d **False.** The magnification produced by a lens is approximately $l/(l + aF)$, where F is the power of the lens, and a is the distance of that lens from the modal point of the eye. In this case, the magnification is over 20%.

    e **False.** In order to see clearly at 33 cm in this device, the patient could accommodate (by significantly more than 3 D, due to the effect of the telescope produced by this lens combination), or the back vertex distance of the spectacles could be increased.

26 a **False.** This level of correction is quite feasible using either rigid corneal, or soft corneal lenses. The highest levels of astigmatism may be corrected using scleral lenses.

    b **False.** Hard contact lenses contain less than 3% water at room temperature.

    c **False.** The tear pump is desirable, even when using a highly gas permeable material, to ensure that epithelial cells and other debris do not collect behind the lens. A tear pump cannot be expected with a thin soft lens, but then lens movement achieves a similar aim.

    d **False.** Only hard lenses are usually able to be re-polished. Gas permeable lenses are usually too thin for this to be achieved, and some designs incorporate surface treatments which would be destroyed in the process. Soft contact lenses cannot usually be re-ground at all.

    e **True.** Steepening the BCOR gives extra positive power, flattening adds minus power.

27 a True. This indicates that the lens centre is vaulting away from the cornea, and is being pressed back by the action of blinking – a characteristic of a tight lens fit.

  b False. A thick lens is best fitted loose to ensure increased tear exchange.

  c False. Base down prisms may be incorporated.

  d False. Soft contact lenses, due to their high comfort, are sometimes the only option when fitting a child with contact lenses.

  e True. At low humidity, soft contact lens materials shrink, leading to tightening of the fit. The effect is most in high water content materials, which often means that such lenses are unsuitable for patients with reduced tear production.

28 a True. To give adequate gas exchange.

  b True. For improved comfort, and good tear exchange.

  c False. Low refractive index would result in increased lens thickness.

  d True. For improved comfort.

  e False. This would produce chromatic aberration in high powers.

29 a True.

  b True.

  c False. More accommodation is required (at a particular distance) for myopes when fitted with contact lenses. The effect increases as the power of the lens increases. For hypermetropes, the situation is reversed.

  d True. Also more vergence is required for myopes.

  e True.

30 a False. Due to the irregular corneal astigmatism.

  b True. Due to the risk of pseudomonas infection associated with diving.

  c False. Due to the inevitable aniseikonia and loss of fusion which would result.

  d True. Due to the child's age, and the optical effect of spectacles.

  e True. Due to the altered tear chemistry associated with this condition which means contact lens wear is usually problematic. There may be a problem if the patient is unable to care for the lens adequately.

31 a **True.**
  b **False.** A high plus lens is convex in shape, and the centre of such a lens will be the thickest point.
  c **True.** Contact lenses are ballasted by incorporating a low amount of prism, which usually sits inferiorly due to the combined action of gravity and the eyelids.
  d **False.** A spherical hard lens will correct corneal astigmatism.
  e **False.** A scleral lens can be divided into the corneal portion, which carries any optical correction, and the haptic portion which rests on the sclera.

32 a **True.** The Dk, or oxygen permeability, of a contact lens material is a measure of the speed with which oxygen passes through an area when subject to a gas pressure gradient (D is the diffusion coefficient and k the solubility of oxygen for the material). For a particular contact lens, therefore, if the gas pressure gradient is increased, the speed of transmission will rise also.
  b **False.** As the lens thickness is increased, the oxygen flux will fall, and as the partial pressure increases, the oxygen flux will increase.
  c **True.**
  d **True.** When fully hydrated, high water content hydrogels allow a high rate of gas exchange.
  e **True.**

33 a **True.**
  b **True.** Causes of spectacle blur include lens overwear, or an inadequate lens fit. It is undesirable, and may discourage patients from removing their contact lenses. Localised oedema of the corneal epithelium is one possible reason for short term blur on removing contact lenses. Spectacle blur is most often seen with hard contact lenses, and hardly ever occurs with soft lenses.
  c **True.**
  d **True.** This effect can be marked with hard (PMMA) contact lenses, and is only minimal with high water content soft lenses. One reason is habituation due to constant corneal stimulation. If there is epithelial oedema, corneal sensitivity will be reduced.
  e **False.** Although a thick soft lens can mask or correct up to 1 D of corneal astigmatism, a thin soft lens will follow the underlying corneal shape. In such cases, a toric soft contact lens or a rigid lens may be required to ensure good vision.

63

34 a True.
   b False. Since PMMA has very low oxygen transmissibility, gas exchange can only take place via the tears, which are "pumped" behind the lens on blinking.
   c True. Silicone contact lenses have very high oxygen transmissibility. The hydrophobic nature of silicone is a drawback for this type of material.
   d True.
   e True. Bifocal contact lenses (to correct presbyopia) have been produced in rigid and soft forms.

35 a True.
   b False. If the patient is refracted using a trial frame, the BVD measurement is essential for calculating contact lens power. Hypermetropes will require a higher contact lens power than spectacles lens power (and vice versa for myopes) due to lens effectivity. The equation for calculating contact lens power is: $Fc = Fs/(1 - dFs)$ where Fc = CL power (dioptres), Fs = spectacle lens power, d = BVD (metres).
   c False. A thick soft contact lens design may give adequate visual acuity under these conditions, and in any case, a soft toric lens could be used. For many patients, a slight blurring of vision in one eye is acceptable where the fellow eye is well corrected.
   d False. More important factors include possible infection risk, and the possible effects of a contact lens on corneal integrity.
   e False. Not necessarily. If a patient is being treated with eye drops and is wearing soft contact lenses, then preservative binding to the lens will be a problem unless non-preserved drops can be prescribed.

36 a False. For a particular back central optic radius, a decrease in diameter will lead to a looser fit, due to corneal shape.
   b False. There is no recommendation which would be suitable for a majority of cases.
   c False. See above. However, PMMA lenses are normally fitted smaller than gas permeable designs to ensure an increased tear exchange.
   d False. In early keratoconus, fitting with a standard contact lens design will result in central corneal touch and mid-peripheral pooling of fluorescein.
   e True.

37 a **False.** When fitting a new wearer, GP lenses offer improved comfort due to the increased lens diameter that it is possible to use compared to PMMA. However, when refitting a long term PMMA wearer with GP lenses, the most common complaint is of discomfort due to a return of corneal sensitivity with GP lenses. Most PMMA and GP contact lens wearers undergo little or no discomfort, and on balance, there is little to separate the different materials on this basis.

   b **False.**

   c **True.**

   d **True.** In a concave lens design, the curvature of the front surface of the optical portion will be less than that of the back surface.

   e **False.** Fenestrations are not required in most GP contact lenses, although they can be used to improve the fit of a lens in exceptional cases.

38 a **True.**

   b **True.** If vision fluctuates with blinking:

> if vision is poor and variable, and momentarily improves on blinking the lens is fitting tight;
> if vision is variable, and clears on staring after a blink, the lens is loose.

   c **True.** Since astigmatism is not well corrected with this design of lens.

   d **False.** This will result in a flatter lens fit.

   e **False.** Since this will tighten the fit.

39 a **False.** This may be an early sign of giant papillary conjunctivitis or some other inflammation.

   b **False.** This is a sign of a lens with a tight fitting edge.

   c **True.**

   d **False.** This is indicative of desiccation of the conjunctiva in these areas, possibly related to contact lens wear, and/or inadequate tear film.

   e **False.** A loose fitting lens will re-centre more slowly than this.

40 a **False.** These lenses usually have a large diameter.

    b **True.** As less handling is required.

    c **False.** As the lenses spend less time soaking in solutions containing preservatives. However, the high water content of such lenses will mean that any chemicals in solutions or the atmosphere can readily bind to the lens.

    d **True.** Due to tear evaporation.

    e **False.** Lenses need to be removed and cleaned and replaced regularly, but can sometimes be renewed at intervals of over six months. In some cases (e.g. infants) very frequent lens renewals may be necessary if fitted with such lenses.

41 a **True.** Monovision refers to the case where one eye is focused for distance viewing, and the other eye is focused for near. This technique works best in the case of low reading additions, but can be disruptive to binocular vision.

    b **True.** Such contact lenses are available, e.g. the Lifestyle GP lens, an aspheric design, where the power gradually changes from distance (centre of lens) to near (edge of lens). The lens relies on decentration during near tasks to position the appropriate section of the lens in front of the pupil.

    c **True.**

    d **True.**

    e **False.** Although such a lens may initially appear to work by increasing the depth of field, the reduced light level would probably render it impractical.

42 a **False.** Such astigmatism is often more accurately corrected with spectacles, although a tolerable result should be possible with contact lenses in most cases.

    b **True.** The corneal irregularity can be compensated for using a rigid contact lens.

    c **True.** Since contact lenses move with the eyes, they avoid the problem of the patient looking through the edge of their spectacle lenses when adopting the face turn.

    d **True.** Contact lenses will result in less minification of the retinal image, and reduced aberrations.

    e **False.** Vision would not be expected to be significantly different in contact lenses or spectacles.

43 a **False.**

b **False.** Fenestrations are occasionally required in scleral designs, to improve tear exchange, and gas exchange, but rarely in corneal designs.

c **False.**

d **False.** A rigid spherical contact lens will correct almost all of the corneal astigmatism due to the effect of the tear lens.

e **False.** In such a case, a spherical soft lens will assume a similar shape to the cornea, and will, therefore, hardly affect the resultant astigmatism.

44 a **True.** GPC can be due to a variety of possible factors, among them are lens deposits (especially protein), lens materials, contact lens edge design, and contact lens solutions.

b **False.** Surfactant is used prior to the rinsing solution.

c **True.**

d **True.**

e **False.** The cystic form of acanthomoeba which may be found in stagnant tap water is resistant to many contact lens solutions.

45 a **False.** They may be used for near as well as distance vision.

b **True.** The Galilean telescope magnifies by increasing the angle subtended by the object at the eye.

c **False.** Convex lenses are used as simple magnifiers.

d **False.** The object is placed just inside the principal focus in a hand-held magnifier.

e **True.** The simple magnifier forms a virtual, magnified image.

46 a **True.** The virtual image increases in size as the object moves closer to the first principal focus of the lens.

b **True.** A high power plano-convex lens which rests directly on the page is used as simple magnifier.

c **True.** A convex cylindrical lens has little or no refractive power in its long axis and high converging power at right-angles to its axis. A lens as is described thus produces vertical magnification of letters, when placed on a line of print.

d **False.**

e **False.**
$$\text{Magnification} = \frac{\text{Dioptric power}}{4}$$

47 a **True.** Fresnel lenses can be used as magnifiers and confer the advantage of reducing thickness and weight.

   b **False.** Base in prisms are used in the loupe.

   c **True.**

   d **False.** A Fresnel lens consists of a thin plastic sheet which has a series of prisms. Spherical aberration will be similar to a conventional spherical lens.

   e **True.** The field of vision is greater where the lens aperture is larger.

48 a **True.** The greater the magnification, the smaller the field of view.

   b **False.** As magnification increases the depth of focus reduces.

   c **False.** Greater magnification requires more illumination.

   d **True.** When the object is at the principal focus of a convex lens, the image is erect, and at infinity.

   e **True.** The image is inverted, diminished, and real.

49 a **False.** In an astronomical telescope both lenses are convex and are separated by the *sum* of their focal lengths.

   b **False.** It consists of a convex objective lens and a concave eye piece lens separated by the difference between the focal lengths.

   c **False.** Forms a virtual image.

   d **True.** With the addition of an auxiliary lens, the Galilean telescope may be used for both near and distance vision.

   e **True.** The combination of a convex and concave lens secures a field relatively free from astigmatism.

50 a **True.**

   b **True.**

   c **False.** The image is virtual and inverted.

   d **True.**

   e **True.** The object of interest (e.g. a stellar body) is well outside the principal focus of the objective.

51 a **False.**
$$\text{Magnification} = \frac{\text{Power of the eye piece}}{\text{Power of the objective}}$$

  b **True.** A concave contact lens can be used as the eye piece of a Galilean telescope.
  c **True.** They can also be incorporated into a bifocal correction.
  d **False.** Base in prisms are used.
  e **True.** An increased field of view is possible when the convex lens is used as the eye piece and the concave lens as the objective.

52 a **True.** Some patients may benefit from reversed contrast, i.e. white print on a black background.
  b **True.** Closed circuit TV allows a high magnification (up to 40 times) without distortion.
  c **False.** The two are equally effective.
  d **True.** The distance Snellen chart may be used closer than 6 m. A Lovie–Bailey chart has the advantage of being able to be used at a greater range of distances.
  e **True.** Such a slit has been seen traditionally by the Eskimos as a protective measure against the UV radiation reflected from the snow.

53 a **True.** Large, low powered magnifiers can be produced which are of light weight.
  b **True.**
  c **True.** The use of Fresnel *prisms* or lenses may cause a reduction in visual acuity due to increased light scatter.
  d **False.**
  e **False.**

54 a **False.** At age 45 a higher amplitude of accommodation than this is normally found.

b **False.** If the patient can use half to two-thirds of her amplitude continuously, then a lens of power $+1\,DS$ or $+1.25\,DS$ is likely to be required for viewing the VDU screen (working distance $= 2\,D$).

c **True.** If the patient can use half to two-thirds of her amplitude continuously, then a lens of power $+2$ or $+2.25\,DS$ is likely to be required for viewing reading material (working distance $= 3\,D$).

d **True.** Although it should be pointed out that they would blur her distance vision.

e **False.** Trifocal lenses would allow this patient to have clear distance vision with the glasses worn, but would result in smaller lens areas for intermediate (VDU) distance and reading, and would add complication and expense.

Clinical refraction

Questions

1 History taking in practical refraction

The following are true:

   a History taking is irrelevant to the final prescription.
   b Previous spectacle wear is important.
   c Lens form is not important.
   d Past ocular history must be enquired after.
   e Hobbies must be enquired after.

2 Regarding initial examination in clinical refraction:

   a It does not include checking visual acuity.
   b It should include a dilated fundal examination.
   c The fellow eye should always be completely occluded while assessing visual acuity.
   d It is helpful to do a direct cover test.
   e If a manifest squint is present, the fixating eye may need occlusion to achieve fixation with the non-dominant eye.

3 Accommodation measured using the RAF rule is usually:

   a The same as that measured by an objective technique, such as retinoscopy.
   b Less than that measured using lenses at 6 m.
   c More binocularly than monocularly.
   d Independent of pupil diameter.
   e Measured using the smallest print the patient can read.

4 The amplitude of accommodation:

    a Refers to maximum amount of accommodation that can be exerted by a patient.

    b Can be measured using the Maddox wing.

    c Is typically of the order of 4 D for a patient aged 60 years.

    d Is best measured using N18 print.

    e Will be greater when measured at 6 m using concave lenses, than if measured using the RAF rule.

5 The AC/A ratio:

    a Might typically have a value of about 3:1 in a patient with no ocular motor abnormality.

    b Will cause symptoms if it is above 5:1.

    c Refers to the amount of accommodation produced by 1Δ of convergence.

    d Cannot be measured in a patient with strabismus.

    e Can be measured at distance or near.

6 Clinical refraction

The following are true:

    a Low power trial lenses should be placed at the back of the trial frame, high power lenses at the front.

    b The examiner should take care not to obstruct the view of the distant fixation object.

    c It is always necessary to use a $+1.5$ DS lens in the trial frame before starting retinoscopy.

    d A "with" movement of the retinoscopy reflex should be corrected with convex lenses.

    e The retinoscopy reflex will move obliquely if there is astigmatism present.

7 Regarding astigmatism in retinoscopy:

a It can be detected on viewing the primary reflex.
b As the point of neutralisation is approached, the axis of a high powered cylinder must only be adjusted a small amount.
c The use of the full cylinder may cause over-correction in adult patients undergoing cycloplegic refraction.
d Findings are often recorded as a power cross.
e It may be determined using spherical lenses alone.

8 Subjective refraction

The following are true:

a Before starting subjective refraction, 1.5 DS should be added to the retinoscopy result.
b Deducting the working distance helps to reduce the cylinder to about one-fourth of its previous value.
c The fellow eye should be occluded.
d The power of the cylinder should be corrected first.
e When verifying the sphere it is necessary to use 0.5 DS increments.

9 Verifying the cylinder, using crossed-cylinder technique:

a The power should be adjusted before the axis.
b The axis is best tested using a circular target.
c The power is best tested using the lowest acuity line.
d The axis should be rechecked if the power is altered.
e If the cylinder is reduced by 1.00 DC, the sphere should be increased by 0.25 DS.

10 In retinoscopy:

a Movement of an aerial image of a reflex from the fundus is judged.
b The speed of the reflex is zero when the refractive error has been neutralised.
c The size of the viewing aperture of the retinoscope affects sensitivity.
d The size of the viewing aperture of the retinoscope does not affect accuracy.
e More accurate results will be achieved by working at a distance of 25 cm, compared to a working distance of 50 cm.

11 When performing retinoscopy:

   a It is not important to be near the visual axis when a low powered lens (e.g. below 1 dioptre) is required.
   b Using a convergent illuminating beam will produce a "with" movement in myopia.
   c Using a beam which is focused in the plane of the patient's pupil will result in a "with" movement.
   d It is best to ask the patient to look directly at the retinoscope light, unless cycloplegia is used.
   e It is always best to occlude the patient's other eye.

12 When performing static retinoscopy:

   a The accommodation of the patient is ideally at the resting point.
   b The power of the working distance lens (in dioptres) is inversely related to the working distance in metres.
   c In patients with a squint, the opposite eye should be occluded.
   d Cycloplegia is required in all patients with squint.
   e The examiner should always sit directly on the visual axis of the patient.

13 Astigmatism:

   a Is termed with-the-rule when a positive cylinder is required at axis 90.
   b Is termed against-the-rule when a negative cylinder is required at axis 45.
   c Of the order of 0.25 to 1.00 DC is not commonly found in the general population.
   d Of 1.00 DC will reduce distance vision to approximately 6/9.
   e Cannot be corrected with contact lenses if above 3 DC.

14 When calculating the near addition:

    a Convex lenses are added to the distance lenses to stimulate accommodation.
    b The approximate value of the near addition for a subject aged 47 is +2.5 DS.
    c An approximate value of the near addition for a subject aged 77 is +2 DS.
    d In general it is advisable to give the maximum plus possible.
    e The patient should be tested reading N5 at their normal reading distance.

15 Measurement of interpupillary distance:

    a Is less important for high prescriptions.
    b Is important in aphakic patients.
    c May be done using corneal light reflexes.
    d May be done using the distance between the nasal limbus of the left eye and the temporal limbus of the right eye.
    e Is approximately 1 mm more than the distance between the visual axes for distance vision.

16 The duochrome test:

    a Gives an estimate of transverse chromatic aberration.
    b Relies upon longitudinal chromatic aberration.
    c Is suitable for use on children as soon as they can read.
    d Is rendered less sensitive by the presence of early nuclear cataract.
    e Can only be used at distance, and not at near.

17 When refracting myopes:

    a They are often intolerant of large changes in their cylindrical axis.
    b They are often intolerant of changes in their lens form.
    c They generally prefer slight under-correction.
    d They may not need a near addition.
    e The duochrome test can be used to prevent over-correction.

18 Regarding spectacle prescription:

    a If a change of cylinder axis is found it should always be prescribed.
    b Pseudophakes often will not tolerate their full cylindrical correction.
    c New bifocal wearers must be warned of difficulty when walking down stairs.
    d Patients appreciate minor changes in their prescription.
    e The lens form must be discussed with the patient.

19 When using cycloplegia for retinoscopy:

    a The mydriasis does not affect the accuracy of the result.
    b The accommodation is only paralysed if the pupil is dilated.
    c The patient's attention should always be directed towards a fixation point at 6 m.
    d The opposite eye should be occluded in all cases.
    e Cycloplegia is only necessary in children.

20 Regarding hypermetropia:

    a It is the most common refractive error in the general population of the UK.
    b Hypermetropia results when the posterior focal length of the eye is longer than the axial length.
    c Absolute hypermetropia is the amount that cannot be overcome by accommodation.
    d Manifest hypermetropia tends to increase with age.
    e Latent hypermetropia tends to decrease with age.

21 Myopia

The following are true:

    a Myopia would be typically termed "axial" in the case of a patient with an axial length of 23 mm.
    b "Axial" myopia is more common than "refractive" myopia in teenage patients.
    c "Index" myopia is caused when the nucleus of the lens undergoes a reduction in refractive index.
    d Myopia can be reduced by flattening the central cornea.
    e The far point of an uncorrected $-2\,DS$ myope is at a theoretical distance of 20 cm.

22 The crossed cylinder:

a Should be used before any attempt is made to correct spherical refractive error.
b Can only be used on patients with VA of at least 6/18.
c Is only used to detect and correct astigmatic refractive error, not spherical refractive error.
d Can only be used with the accommodation relaxed, or paralysed to check astigmatic error.
e Result can be affected by pupil size.

23 A patient with 1.50 dioptre of with-the-rule astigmatism:

a Will usually complain of vision which is more blurred at distance than at near.
b Will have a blurred retinal image for objects at all distances.
c Will require a correcting lens with positive axis vertical.
d Cannot be corrected with contact lenses.
e Would be expected to have an uncorrected VA of no better than 6/18.

24 When prescribing spectacles:

a It is not necessary to note the BVD unless the prescription is above 8 DS.
b The optical centres of spectacle lenses should always be at the patient's IPD.
c A maximum of 2 D of anisometropia can be tolerated.
d Plastic lenses are the lens of choice for children.
e Glass lenses are always heavier than plastic lenses of the same prescription.

25 When prescribing spectacles:

    a Attention need only be paid to lens centration when the lens power exceeds 4 D in any one meridian.

    b A decentration of 5 mm UP on a + 1 DS lens will produce a prismatic effect of 0.5ΔUP.

    c A prismatic error of 0.5ΔUP would be expected to produce significant symptoms in the majority of patients.

    d Photochromics should not be prescribed to children.

    e For a lens power of − 3 DS, polycarbonate lenses are usually heavier than glass lenses.

26 A 71-year-old patient has VA of 6/18 R and L due to age-related macular degeneration:

    a This patient could be expected to read N6 print with a + 3 D reading addition.

    b For watching television, this patient would most benefit from a pair of 2 × telescopes mounted in a spectacle frame, as this would give an equivalent 6/6 acuity.

    c A pair of 4 × telescopes would be useful for shopping.

    d This patient should be advised that their vision will make night driving difficult, but that driving in bright sunlight will be relatively easy.

    e A + 12 D magnifying lens would give about 2 × or 3 × magnification for reading.

27 A 60-year-old emmetropic patient is prescribed pilocarpine drops in both eyes for the treatment of glaucoma. The following can be expected:

    a Reading without glasses is possible due to miosis.

    b Distance vision is blurred, due to excess accommodation.

    c Distance vision is blurred, due to miosis.

    d Distance vision is clearer than previously.

    e When entering a darkened environment from a light environment, vision is immediately clear, as the retina has been previously protected from light adaptation by the miosis.

28 Amblyopia:

a May be tested for using neutral density filters.
b Tends to have a greater degree of crowding phenomenon compared to the normal eye.
c May be strabismic.
d May be caused by congenital ptosis.
e Does not occur in anisometropia.

29 Cover tests:

a The monocular (or direct) cover test only detects heterophorias.
b The alternate cover test only elicits heterotropias.
c In the direct cover test, if covering the right eye causes the left eye to move nasally to take up fixation, the patient has a left exotropia.
d If the alternate prism cover test is done before the direct prism cover test it may be impossible to differentiate between a phoria and a tropia.
e The prism cover test is used to measure total deviation.

30 Dissociated image tests

The following are true:

a The Maddox wing dissociates the eyes at distance.
b Risley prisms are used to measure phorias and fusional vergence amplitude.
c When the Maddox rod cylinders are horizontal, the image seen is also horizontal.
d With the Maddox rod in the vertical orientation in front of the right eye, the left eye sees a horizontal red line.
e Maddox rod may be used to measure cyclotropia.

79

31 Orthoptic tests

The following are true:

a The Hess chart involves the use of a plane mirror.
b The Lees screen is tested with the patient wearing red–green filter goggles.
c The Worth four-dot, Bagolini lenses and the after-image tests detect anomalous retinal correspondence.
d The synoptophore may be used to detect anomalous retinal correspondence and amblyopia, and to grade binocular vision.
e The third grade of binocular vision is fusion, according to Worth's classification.

32 Stereopsis tests

The following are true:

a The Titmus test includes vectographs viewed with red–green goggles.
b The Worth four-dot test detects stereopsis.
c The TNO test covers a range of stereoacuity from 480 to 15 seconds of arc.
d The Lang stereotest gives a gross indication of stereoacuity.
e The Frisby test requires the use of polarising glasses.

33 The expected value for visual acuity of a cooperative 5-year-old child would be:

a 6/18 Kay pictures.
b 6/12 Sheridan Gardiner single letters.
c 6/9 Sheridan Gardiner single letters.
d 6/12 Snellen chart.
e 6/6 Snellen chart.

34 Regarding refraction of children:

   a Cycloplegia is always necessary to obtain an accurate refraction.
   b A full correction is often not tolerated in high myopia.
   c It is always necessary to deduct 1 D sphere to compensate for a cycloplegic refraction.
   d Myopia should be corrected in the presence of large exophoria or exotropia.
   e Uncorrected anisometropic hypermetropia results in amblyopia of the less hypermetropic eye.

35 Regarding heterophorias:

   a Myopia may be associated with esophoria or esotropia.
   b Myopia may be associated with exophoria or exotropia.
   c Hypermetropia is usually associated with exophoria or exotropia.
   d The distribution of phorias in the general population follows a normal distribution.
   e A patient with a manifest squint cannot have a phoria.

36 In patients with congenital nystagmus:

   a Retinoscopy is impossible if the patient cannot keep their eyes still.
   b The refractive error can be expected to show positive astigmatism, axis vertical.
   c Base in prisms often improve visual acuity.
   d Spectacles should only be required if the prescription is above 4 D.
   e Contact lenses offer no advantages.

37 If, following retinoscopy, a patient's acuity is 6/18:

   a Approximately 1 D of spherical error would be anticipated.
   b Approximately 1 D of cylindrical error would be anticipated.
   c The pinhole test will indicate whether there is any residual refractive error present.
   d The crossed-cylinder test should be the first step of the subjective refraction.
   e The pinhole test cannot be performed if the patient has a manifest strabismus, as the fovea will not be aligned with the pinhole.

38 If a 6-year-old patient has a manifest strabismus measuring 20 PD esotropia:

    a One eye should be occluded during retinoscopy.

    b Cycloplegia should be used to obtain the most accurate objective result.

    c The minimum positive power that gives good distance acuity should be prescribed.

    d The pinhole test cannot usually be performed with a child of this age.

    e The Snellen letter chart cannot usually be used with a child of this age.

39 A 52-year-old VDU operator is -1.00 DS myopic. His accommodative amplitude measures as 2 D. Which of the following prescriptions is appropriate for this patient?

    a Bifocals, -1.00 DS with a $+3.00$ DS addition for reading at 33 cm.

    b Single vision lenses, $+2.50$ DS for reading at 33 cm.

    c Single vision lenses, $+2.00$ DS for reading a VDU screen at 50 cm.

    d Bifocals, plano with a $+1.00$ DS addition for reading a VDU screen at 50 cm, and reading at 33 cm.

    e Trifocals, a -1.00 DS, intermediate addition $+1.00$ DS, near addition $+2.00$ DS for distance, reading the VDU at 50 cm and reading at 33 cm.

40 When measuring the visual field of patients wearing spectacles that correct their refractive errors:

    a The blind spot (due to the optic nerve head) is larger and closer to fixation in the case of a hypermetrope, compared to an emmetrope.

    b The blind spot is smaller and closer to fixation in the case of a myope, compared to an emmetrope.

    c The blind spot appears larger, but in the same position, in the case of a hypermetrope, compared to a myope.

    d The blind spot is smaller and further from fixation in a myope compared to a hypermetrope.

    e The blind spot is unaffected in the case of an astigmat, compared to an emmetrope.

41 The following statements are true:

    a The far point of an emmetrope is at infinity.

    b The far point of a hypermetrope is nearer than that of a myope.

    c The near point of a myope, expressed in dioptres, is equal to the distance refractive error.

    d The difference between the far and near points, expressed in dioptres, is equal to the amplitude of accommodation.

    e If a patient's refractive error is wrongly prescribed, the distance between the near and far points, in dioptres, is not equal to the amplitude of accommodation.

42 The following techniques are used to refine the spherical component of the refraction:

    a Block and fan.

    b Duochrome.

    c Fixation disparity tests.

    d Binocular balancing.

    e Dynamic crossed cylinder.

Clinical refraction

Answers

1 a **False.** History is important to ascertain the patient's age, occupation, and special requirements.
  b **True.**
  c **False.** Myopes are especially intolerant to changes in lens form.
  d **True.**
  e **True.**

2 a **False.** Visual acuity should be measured for near and distance, both unaided and with current spectacles.
  b **False.** This should normally be done at the end of the refraction.
  c **False.** In patients with nystagmus a high plus lens should be used as complete occlusion sometimes increases nystagmus and may reduce acuity.
  d **True.** This detects manifest squint.
  e **True.**

3 a **False.** Because of the depth of field of the eye at near, accommodation appears greater when measured subjectively than objectively.
  b **False.** Because of proximal accommodation effects, patients can more readily accommodate for an object at near.
  c **True.**
  d **False.** Pupil constriction leads to an increase in depth of field.
  e **True.**

4 a **True.**

  b **False.** The Maddox wing is used to measure near ocular motor balance.

  c **False.** A patient of this age would normally have less accommodation available.

  d **False.** It is best measured using the smallest print the patient can read, so that blur is easily recognised.

  e **False.** The lack of proximal cues (and if carried out binocularly, vergence accommodation) invariably means that the amplitude is less when measured using a distance target.

5 a **True.** Quoted "normal" values are of the order of 3:1.

  b **False.** High or low AC/A ratios can be present without symptoms.

  c **False.** The AC/A ratio is a measure of the amount of convergence (in prism dioptres) produced by 1 D of accommodation.

  d **False.**

  e **True.**

6 a **False.** High power lenses should be placed posteriorly.

  b **True.** If the examiner gets in the way, the patient may start to accommodate.

  c **False.**

  d **True.**

  e **True.**

7 a **True.** Astigmatism will cause the retinoscopy reflex to move obliquely.

  b **True.** The angle of misalignment of the reflex is much greater than the angle of misalignment of the cylindrical lens in this case.

  c **True.** This is due to the fact that most patients will not tolerate their full cylindrical correction.

  d **True.**

  e **True.**

8 a **False.** The working distance should be deducted.

  b **False.** Power of the working distance lens is spherical, and does not affect the cylinder.

  c **True.**

  d **False.** The power of the sphere is the initial correction.

  e **False.** If visual acuity is good, smaller increments (0.25 DS) can be used.

9 a **False.** The axis should be checked before the power.

  b **True.**

  c **True.**

  d **True.**

  e **False.** The sphere increases by 0.5 D.

10 a **True.**

  b **False.** At neutralisation, the speed of the reflex is so high that its direction cannot be judged. The light from the patient's pupil appears to flash on and off when the retinoscope is moved.

  c **True.** A larger viewing aperture increases sensitivity at the cost of accuracy – in other words, with a small aperture, a refractive error is less easily detected, but neutralisation is achieved with more certainty.

  d **False.**

  e **False.** Except in the case of a dim reflex (e.g. due to small pupils, or media opacities, when sitting close is the only option), accuracy generally increases as working distance increases.

11 a **False.** Errors may occur in any patient if retinoscopy is not performed near the visual axis.

  b **True.**

  c **False.** This will result in a "neutral" response in all patients.

  d **False.** In the absence of cycloplegia, this will result in accommodation, and a difficult view due to pupillary constriction.

  e **False.** This is only necessary for patients with strabismus. Otherwise, it is best to leave the patient with both eyes open to help relax accommodation.

12 a **False.** Ideally, no accommodation should be exerted by the patient. The resting point of the accommodation system occurs at a distance of approximately 50–100 cm but this varies with factors such as refractive state, age, previous viewing distance etc.

   b **True.**

   c **True.** So that the visual axis of the eye being worked on is not deviated.

   d **False.** Cycloplegia is only required to control accommodation and would not usually be required in an adult patient with a squint.

   e **False.** In cycloplegic refraction, the examiner should be directly in line with the patient's visual axis. When cycloplegia is not used it is better to sit slightly off the patient's visual axis to avoid stimulation of accommodation and pupil constriction.

13 a **True.**

   b **False.**

   c **False.**

   d **True.**

   e **False.**

14 a **False.** Concave lenses are added.

   b **False.** An addition of around $+1\,DS$ is more suitable for most patients of this age.

   c **False.** $+2.5\,DS$ would probably be required (at least).

   d **False.** Generally patients will not tolerate too high a near addition.

   e **True.**

15 a **False.** Decentration causes unwanted prismatic effects especially in high powered lenses.

   b **True.** See above.

   c **True.**

   d **True.**

   e **True.** This is the actual measurement required for making spectacles.

16 a **False.** The effect of *transverse* chromatic aberration on vision would be to produce coloured fringes at edges.

   b **True.** The effect of longitudinal chromatic aberration is a dependence of focal length upon the wavelength of light used. Thus, for the eye, approximately 0.50 DS separates the red and green foci.

   c **False.** The duochrome test becomes unreliable if the patient has very active accommodation, and this is often the case for young children.

   d **True.** Due to the yellowing of the lens associated with nuclear cataract, patients may see the red light as *brighter* than the green, and may therefore tend to report the red as being clearer.

   e **False.** When used at near, letters on the green background are seen more clearly than those on the red background, in most cases.

17 a **True.**

   b **True.**

   c **True.** This means that they do not have to accommodate for the distance.

   d **True.**

   e **True.** The myopic patient should see the red letters more clearly to ensure under-correction.

18 a **False.** Only change the axis of the cylinder if the patient is symptomatic, especially in a myope.

   b **False.**

   c **True.**

   d **False.** There is no need to give a patient new glasses for a minor change in prescription unless there is a very good reason.

   e **True.** Some patients are intolerant of varifocal glasses etc. So their requirements must be taken into consideration.

19 a **False.** The large pupil will reduce accuracy.

   b **False.** The mydriasis lags behind the cycloplegic effect.

   c **False.** The patient should fixate on the retinoscope.

   d **False.** This is only necessary if the patient has a squint.

   e **False.** Cycloplegia may be needed for adults, e.g. if there is poor cooperation or ciliary spasm.

20 a **True.**
  b **True.**
  c **True.**
  d **False.**
  e **True.**

21 a **False.**
  b **True.**
  c **False.**
  d **True.**
  e **False.** 50 cm.

22 a **False.** If the spherical error is not corrected prior to the use of the cross cylinder the technique will be less sensitive.
  b **False.** In cases with reduced VA, a higher power crossed cylinder will often produce a result, but the sensitivity of the test is reduced.
  c **False.** Spherical error is assessed in the dynamic crossed cylinder test.
  d **False.** To ensure that the circle of least confusion is on the retina, it is better if accommodation is active.
  e **True.** Sensitivity can be reduced by small pupils.

23 a **True.** Although astigmatism theoretically reduces image quality at all distances, the increased depth of field of the eye at near means that symptoms are worse at distance.
  b **True.**
  c **True.**
  d **False.**
  e **False.**

24 a **False.** The BVD should always be measured and recorded if one meridian of the prescription is 6 D or more. It is good practice to do this for powers of 4 D.

   b **False.** This depends on the prescription. For low powers, a negligible prismatic effect is induced by slight decentration. In cases where a prism is prescribed, decentration is often employed to deliberately create a prismatic effect.

   c **False.** Much higher levels of anisometropia than this may be tolerated in practice, although there is a large individual variation between patients.

   d **True.**

   e **False.** For high minus prescriptions, for example, the lighter lens may be a glass lens of high refractive index.

25 a **False.** Lens centration can be critical on lenses of a lower power than this, especially in the vertical direction.

   b **True.**

   c **False.** For the majority of patients, this amount of vertical prism would be tolerated without problems. However, the patient may be aware of some initial mild discomfort while adapting to the glasses.

   d **False.** Glass spectacle lenses which are not toughened or laminated pose a risk for children (and indeed, all patients). However, photochromic lenses are available in toughened glass, and plastics. The toughened glass photochromic lenses typically react more slowly, and with a smaller range of tints than the non-toughened glass type, whilst the latest plastic photochromics react quickly, and with a wide range. Cost may be an issue.

   e **False.**

26 a **False.** Reading acuity can be roughly estimated from distance acuity as follows: 6/(X) should result in N(X/2). However, in the case of macula disorders, the reading acuity is typically reduced more than the distance acuity.

   b **False.** Although fine in principle, telescopes are rarely beneficial for a task such as television, where a larger screen or reduced viewing distance is possible.

   c **False.** Because they result in a restricted field of view, and partially disable the VOR, telescopes grossly affect mobility.

   d **False.** This patient should be advised that their vision is below the legal standard for driving in the UK.

   e **True.**

27 a **True.** Due to the increased depth of field.
   b **False.** A patient of this age cannot be expected to have useful reserves of accommodation.
   c **False.**
   d **False.**
   e **False.** A mobile pupil dramatically speeds up dark adaptation, and a patient on pilocarpine can be expected to notice that vision is much worse under these circumstances.

28 a **True.** Neutral density filters are used to distinguish between organic and amblyopic causes of reduced visual acuity. If use of neutral density filters does not make a significant difference to the visual acuity, the defect is likely to be amblyopia. If there is a significant decrease in acuity, the cause is more likely to be organic.
   b **True.** The crowding phenomenon describes a reduction in visual acuity when reading a row of letters rather than single letters. The presence of contours next to the letter being read reduces visual acuity in both normal and amblyopic subjects.
   c **True.** Strabismus may result in suppression of the deviated eye causing amblyopia.
   d **True.** Complete unilateral ptosis is associated with severe deprivational amblyopia.
   e **False.** Anisometropia commonly leads to amblyopia in the *more* hypermetropic eye.

29 a **False.** The monocular (or direct) cover test identifies heterotropias and heterophorias.
   b **False.** The alternate cover test also elicits the maximum angle of heterophorias.
   c **True.**
   d **True.** In some patients, binocular vision is so disrupted by performing the alternate cover test that the phoria becomes manifest. In such cases therefore, it is important to perform the direct cover first.
   e **True.** The prism cover test measures total deviation (latent plus manifest).

30 a **False.** The Maddox wing is used at 33 cm.
   b **True.** A Risley prism is a prism made up of two prisms, usually of around 15 D power, which are counter-rotated. The resultant power varies from 0 to 30 D.
   c **False.** The linear image seen is at right-angles to the axis of the cylinders; in this case it is vertical.
   d **False.** With the Maddox rod in the vertical orientation in front of the right eye, the *right* eye sees a horizontal red line and the left eye should see a white spot.
   e **True.**

31 a **False.** The Hess chart uses red–green goggles to dissociate the eyes. It maps out the range of movement of each eye and identifies paretic muscles.
   b **False.** The Lees screen is similar to the Hess test but a plane mirror is used to dissociate the eyes.
   c **True.** Anomalous retinal correspondence occurs when a deviating eye fixates with an area outside the foveola.
   d **True.** The synoptophore is also used to assess strabismus.
   e **False.** According to Worth's classification there are three grades of the degree of binocular vision present; simultaneous perception; fusion; stereoscopic vision.

32 a **False.** The Titmus test is viewed with polaroid glasses. It tests stereoacuity from 3000 to 40 seconds of arc.
   b **False.** The Worth four-dot test detects suppression and anomalous retinal correspondence.
   c **True.** The TNO test consists of computer generated random dot anaglyphs viewed through red–green spectacles.
   d **True.** The stereoacuity range is of the order of 1200 to 550 seconds of arc.
   e **False.** The Frisby test is in itself three-dimensional and does not require polaroid or coloured spectacles.

33 a **False.**
   b **False.**
   c **False.**
   d **False.**
   e **True.**

34 a False. The Mohindra technique of refracting children in a blackened room allows the accurate refraction of children without cycloplegia. Older children may not require cycloplegia.

  b True. It is important to correct high myopia as early as possible as it may cause retarded development. However, a prescription which is one or two dioptres less than the full correction may be much better tolerated.

  c False. In general, when a patient has a heterotropia, the maximum plus prescription is given and in this case the cycloplegic correction would not be made.

  d True. Correction of the myopia in these cases helps to stimulate accommodation and convergence.

  e False. Anisometropic hypermetropia may result in amblyopia of the *more* hypermetropic eye (and occasionally of the less hypermetropic eye).

35 a True.

  b True.

  c False. Hypermetropia is usually associated with esophoria or esotropia.

  d False. The distribution shows considerable kurtosis, with a large peak around orthophoria.

  e False. In the presence of ARC, a patient with a squint can have a co-existing phoria.

36 a False. Retinoscopy will be made easier if the patient can look in the direction of their null zone. However, it is still possible to judge the refractive error. Such patients often have high levels of WTR astigmatism.

  b True.

  c False. Base out prisms to stimulate convergence may improve VA in some cases.

  d False. Particularly in children, correcting the refractive error should be tried, as this may reduce the "effort to see", and result in an improvement of the nystagmus waveform.

  e False. Contact lenses move with the eyes, and therefore offer a slight optical improvement due to the CN movements, and in cases of abnormal head posture associated with nystagmus. Contact lenses may also reduce CN amplitude.

37 a **True.** In the presence of a typical pupil of 3–4 mm diameter, 1 D of spherical error can be expected to reduce VA to 6/12 or 6/18.

 b **False.** In the presence of a typical pupil of 3–4 mm diameter, 2 D of cylindrical error can be expected to reduce VA to 6/12 or 6/18.

 c **True.**

 d **False.** The spherical component of the refraction must be corrected before the crossed cylinder test is performed.

 e **False.** The pinhole can still be used in the presence of a manifest strabismus.

38 a **True.** Otherwise, there is a danger of being a long way off the visual axis during retinoscopy.

 b **True.** Although good results may be obtained using non-cycloplegic retinoscopy in a child of this age, active accommodation will probably render the technique inaccurate.

 c **False.** This will encourage accommodation (and accommodative convergence), exacerbating the strabismus.

 d **False.**

 e **False.**

39 a **False.**

 b **False.**

 c **False.**

 d **True.**

 e **True.**

40 a **False.** Through a plus lens, the blind spot appears closer to fixation, and all isopters appear smaller.

 b **False.** Through a minus lens, the blind spot appears farther from fixation, and magnified in size.

 c **False.** Compared to the myope, the blind spot of the hypermetrope is smaller and closer to fixation.

 d **False.** The blind spot is larger and further from fixation in a myope compared to a hypermetrope.

 e **False.** The blind spot is affected due to the meridional magnification of a cylindrical spectacle lens.

41 a True.
   b False.
   c False.
   d True.
   e False.

42 a False.
   b True.
   c False.
   d True.
   e True.

Instruments

Questions

1 Changes in refractive error

The following are true:

a Children tend to become less hypermetropic in the first few years of life.
b Blunt trauma may cause a sudden change in refractive error.
c Nucleosclerosis causes a myopic shift.
d Diabetic hyperglycaemia may cause a sudden myopic trend.
e Retinal detachment surgery may result in a myopic change.

2 The following instruments use captoptric images:

a Placidos disc.
b The pachometer.
c The indirect ophthalmoscope.
d The direct ophthalmoscope.
e The Javal–Schiotz keratometer.

3 The Scheiner principle:

a Describes the use of a single pinhole to improve vision.
b Is used in the manufacture of all automated refractors.
c Is a zonal focus method of refraction.
d Is used in infrared optometers.
e Helps ascertain the axis of astigmatism.

4 Infrared optometers:

    a Are objective.
    b Use a fixation target to encourage maximum accommodation.
    c Provide a different refraction to that in visible light.
    d May be unreliable if the subject has pupil abnormalities.
    e Are inaccurate with vision less than 6/18.

5 Regarding new developments in automated refraction:

    a Photographic methods are more accurate than clinical refraction.
    b Laser speckle pattern refraction is objective.
    c The Humphrey Vision Analyser employs a convex mirror in which the patient views targets.
    d The Humphrey Vision Analyser uses Alvarez variable power lenses.
    e The Humphrey Vision Analyser is useful for young children.

6 The focimeter:

    a Measures the vertex power of a lens.
    b Cannot measure prismatic power.
    c Contains a viewing telescope.
    d Has a concave collimating lens.
    e Can be used to measure contact lens power.

7 The Galilean telescope:

    a Contains two convex lenses.
    b The two lenses are separated by the difference in their focal lengths.
    c May be used as an LVA for near and distance.
    d May reduce depth of focus.
    e Enables rapid scanning of information due to the large field of view.

8 The focimeter

The following are true:

a The axes as well as the powers of an astigmatic lens may be measured with a focimeter.

b The spectacle lens must be mounted with the front surface of the lens against the rest to measure back vertex power.

c The target is moved through a distance directly proportional to the power of the lens.

d Light entering the viewing telescope is diverging.

e The test lens lies at the principal focus of the collimating lens.

9 The indirect ophthalmoscope:

a Is used with a powerful concave lens, usually 13 D or 20 D.

b Light refracted by the condensing lens forms a virtual image between the lens and the observer.

c Is advantageous in viewing myopic fundi compared with the direct ophthalmoscope.

d The field of view is limited by the observer's pupil and the aperture of the condensing lens.

e Presbyopic observers may need to use their own glasses in addition to the viewing piece.

10 When using the indirect ophthalmoscope:

a The field of illumination is largest in a hypermetropic subject.

b The pupil size of the subject limits the field of illumination.

c Light from a point in the pupillary plane of the subject is focused by the condensing lens in the pupillary plane of the observer.

d The image seen is laterally but not vertically inverted.

e The field of view is up to four times larger than with the direct ophthalmoscope.

11 The indirect ophthalmoscope:

a Does not give a binocular view of the fundus.
b Has lenses in the eyepiece.
c Produces greater magnification with a $+13$ D lens compared to a $+20$ D lens.
d Can be used with a teaching mirror.
e Has a more powerful light source than the direct ophthalmoscope.

12 The indirect and direct ophthalmoscopes

The following are true:

a The 28 D lens is useful in paediatric ophthalmology.
b In myopes the image size increases as the lens is moved away from the eye.
c The direct is the instrument of choice for examining retinal detachments.
d The direct produces greater magnification than the indirect.
e The direct produces an inverted image.

13 Regarding the direct ophthalmoscope:

a It can be used to view the anterior segment.
b It contains a plane mirror with a hole in it permitting the observer to view the subject.
c The field of view does not depend upon the patient's refractive error.
d Mydriasis enhances the field of view.
e The field of view decreases with close proximity to the subject.

14 When using the direct ophthalmoscope:

a The magnification varies with the refractive error of the subject.
b In the case of a hypermetropic patient and an emmetropic observer, the observer should accommodate or use a correcting lens to focus the image.
c Aphakic eyes produce a magnified image compared to emmetropic eyes.
d Marked astigmatism cannot be negated by adjusting the lenses.
e The magnification is 15 times.

15 Regarding the retinoscope:

    a It consists of a mirror with a central aperture and a light source.
    b With a condensing lens at the top, the effect is that of a plane mirror.
    c It is usually used with the plane mirror effect.
    d As the neutralisation point is reached, the reflex slows down.
    e An image of the illuminated retina is formed at the patient's far point.

16 In measuring corneal curvature:

    a The central 4 mm of the cornea is assumed to be spherical.
    b There are two types of keratometer: Javal–Schiotz and Placidos disc.
    c The Von Helmholtz keratometer uses a fixed image size.
    d The Javal–Schiotz keratometer uses two rotating glass plates to double the image.
    e The Von Helmholtz keratometer can be used to measure astigmatism.

17 The Placidos disc:

    a Is a convex disc with concentric black and white rings.
    b Has a central aperture in which a concave lens is mounted.
    c Requires illumination positioned behind the observer's head.
    d Measures corneal curvature.
    e Can be used to detect keratoconus.

18 The keratometer:

    a Uses image doubling to overcome movements of the patient's eye.
    b Is also called the ophthalmometer.
    c May be used to measure the axes of astigmatism of the cornea.
    d Uses the second Purkinje–Sanson image.
    e Is important in contact lens fitting.

19 The keratometer

The following are true:

a   The Javal–Schiotz keratometer has mires designed such that each step of the mire is equivalent to 2D of corneal power.
b   The image of the mires is magnified and real.
c   The central 10 mm of corneal diameter is measured.
d   The image is doubled using a Risley prism.
e   The dioptric power of the cornea is inversely related to its radius.

20 The compound microscope:

a   Gives a magnified view of a distant object.
b   Is used with the keratometer, pachometer, and tonometer.
c   Contains a Porro prism.
d   Has a convex objective and a concave eye piece.
e   Has an eye piece which acts as a loupe.

21 When using the compound microscope:

a   The object to be studied is placed just outside the anterior focal point.
b   A real, inverted, diminished image forms behind the objective lens.
c   The image formed by the objective falls close to the principal focal plane of the eye piece lens.
d   The final image is vertically and horizontally inverted.
e   The specular microscope is a modified form of the compound microscope.

22 Regarding the slit lamp biomicroscope:

a   It contains two compound microscopes separated by an angle of 20 degrees.
b   Specular reflection is useful for viewing the corneal endothelium.
c   Retro-illumination may be used to detect abnormalities of the anterior capsule.
d   The blue filter is useful for viewing the vitreous.
e   It may be used with the illumination column tilted.

23 The slit lamp

The following are true:

a The slit lamp is a high-powered telescope.
b The microscope and light system have a common focal plane.
c There is a short distance between the microscope and the subject's eye.
d Sclerotic scatter involves directing the slit beam at the edge of the limbus, causing the whole limbal area to glow.
e The green filter is useful for viewing the vitreous.

24 Regarding fundus viewing lenses:

a The Hruby lens is a plano-convex lens of strength $+58$ D.
b The Hruby lens forms a real image anterior to the retina.
c The 90 D lens forms a real image within the focal range of the slit lamp.
d The 78 D gives a larger field of view than the 90 D.
e The fundus viewing contact lens which is used in vitrectomies is plano-concave.

25 Regarding fundus viewing lenses:

a The Hruby lens is best used with the lens close to the subject's eye.
b The Hruby lens is held with its concave surface towards the eye.
c The Goldmann contact lenses have a higher refractive index than the eye.
d The central zone of the 3 mirror and gonioscopy lenses are unsuitable for viewing the fundus.
e The 90 and 78 D are powerful concave lenses.

26 Regarding tonometry:

a The Goldmann is an indentation tonometer.
b Applanation tonometry is based on the Imbert Fick principle.
c The IOP is read when the area of corneal contact is 3.06 mm diameter.
d The Perkins is a portable tonometer of similar principle to the Schiotz tonometer.
e The tonometer head contains two base out prisms.

27 Regarding the applanation tonometer:

    a When used correctly, the effect of surface tension and the rigidity of the cornea negate each other.

    b The applanation head is mounted on a spring loaded lever.

    c The air-puff tonometer is based on the Imbert Fick principle.

    d The air-puff tonometer gives identical readings to the Goldmann tonometer.

    e The inner edges of the fluorescein meniscus define the area of contact.

28 The pachometer

The following are true:

    a The pachometer uses Purkinje–Sanson image III to measure corneal thickness.

    b Image doubling in the Jaeger pachometer is by means of a special eye piece.

    c The Maurice–Giardine pachometer splits the incident light using a perspex plate.

    d When using the Maurice–Giardine pachometer a perspex plate is rotated until the two corneal surfaces are superimposed.

    e The Haag–Streit pachometer is used by rotating a plate until the anterior and posterior corneal surfaces are juxtaposed.

29 Pachometers:

    a Can be used to measure anterior chamber depth.

    b Use Purkinje–Sanson images I and II to measure corneal thickness.

    c Use Purkinje–Sanson images III and IV to measure anterior chamber depth.

    d May be of the Javal–Schiotz or Von Helmholtz type.

    e Can be used to measure axial length.

30 PAM scanning:

 a Allows assessment of macular function in the presence of a media opacity.
 b Projects an acuity chart on the retina through a small aperture.
 c Requires a clear window in the media.
 d Overcomes most refractive errors.
 e Cannot be relied upon in the presence of a mature cataract.

31 The following are true:

 a Scanning laser ophthalmoscopy (SLO) uses infra-red radiation to obtain images of the fundus.
 b A-scan ultrasonography measures axial length.
 c A-scan uses a non-focused beam.
 d B-scan is a real time kinetic scan.
 e Contact and immersion scans are terms relevant to an A-scan.

32 The fundus camera:

 a Separates illumination and observation beams.
 b Forms the aerial image anterior to the holed mirror.
 c Is used in fluorescein angiography.
 d Incorporates filters.
 e Forms a real image.

33 Regarding zoom systems:

 a They allow a continuous adjustment of power.
 b Zoom systems are used in operating microscopes.
 c In compensated systems the image is at the same position relative to the front element.
 d Uncompensated systems are best suited for photography.
 e Mechanically compensated zoom systems move the rear element.

34 Regarding the methods for estimating visual potential in the presence of opacities of the optical media:

a   The blue field entoptic test is a test of macular function.

b   In the contra-light test, visual acuity is reduced due to the effect of glare.

c   Noise charts do not reveal the effect of neural damage, only loss of contrast sensitivity due to poor optical quality.

d   Oscillatory movement detection thresholds (OMDTs) are a hyperacuity task.

e   Oscillatory movement detection thresholds are reduced more by opacities of the media than by macula dysfunction.

35 Considering the optical design of ophthalmoscopes:

a   When performing direct ophthalmoscopy, an upright, virtual image of the fundus of the patient is viewed.

b   Indirect ophthalmoscopy produces a real image of the fundus of the patient.

c   The direct ophthalmoscope gives no information as to the refractive error of the patient.

d   When performing indirect ophthalmoscopy, the lens used must be held at a distance equal to its focal length from the cornea of the patient.

e   In the scanning laser ophthalmoscope, the purpose of the confocal aperture is to significantly reduce the brightness of objects outside the focal plane of the instrument.

Instruments

Answers

1 a **True.** The myopic change occurs with general growth.
  b **True.** Blunt trauma commonly causes a transient change in refractive error.
  c **True.**
  d **True.** In diabetes, the changes in refraction occur bilaterally and suddenly – myopia is associated with hyperglycaemia and hypermetropia with hypoglycaemia.
  e **True.** The use of encircling bands elongates the axial length, inducing myopia.

2 a **True.**
  b **False.**
  c **False.**
  d **False.**
  e **True.**

3 a **False.**
  b **False.** Other designs include the indirect ophthalmoscope principle, the coincidence optometer principle, and designs based on the retinoscope.
  c **True.**
  d **True.**
  e **True.** The axis of astigmatism can be found by rotating a Scheiner disc and asking the patient to report when the spots are maximally separated.

4 a **True.** The instrument itself senses the end-point of refraction.
   b **False.** The target is designed to encourage relaxation of accommodation.
   c **True.** This is because of chromatic aberration of the eye and because infra-red light is reflected from different retinal layers to visible light.
   d **True.** For example, pupil distortion or miosed pupils may give rise to errors.
   e **True.**

5 a **False.** They have a limited role in screening for ametropia.
   b **False.** It is a subjective method which is sensitive to 0.25 DS.
   c **False.** The mirror is concave.
   d **True.** Each Alvarez lens unit consists of two lenses with optical surfaces designed to give a variable focal length when combined.
   e **False.** It requires a skilled operator and a cooperative patient.

6 a **True.**
   b **False.** The prismatic power can be measured. The decentration of the lens is measured against the cross lines of the graticule. The graticule is calibrated at 1 PD intervals and this enables calculation of prismatic power.
   c **True.** A focimeter consists of a collimating lens and a viewing telescope. Light from an illuminated object passes through the lens to be measured, and the collimating lens is positioned to produce parallel light, which is viewed with the telescope. The position of the collimating lens depends on the power of the lens to be measured.
   d **False.** This is a converging lens.
   e **True.**

7 a **False.** The Galilean telescope consists of a convex lens as the objective and a concave lens as the eye piece.
   b **True.** This is true when the lens is focused for optical infinity. Due to the fact that the concave lens has its second focal point behind the lens, a Galilean telescope is less bulky than an astronomical telescope.
   c **True.** Such telescopes can have a large range of focus.
   d **True.** The depth of focus reduces as magnification increases.
   e **False.** Telescopes have a small field of view, particularly Galilean telescopes.

8 a **True.**
  b **False.** The spectacle must be mounted with the back surface against the rest, so that the back vertex power may be measured.
  c **True.**
  d **False.** Light entering the telescope is collimated (parallel).
  e **True.**

9 a **False.** A powerful convex lens is used to produce an aerial image of the fundus.
  b **False.** The aerial image is real.
  c **True.** Due to the larger field of view with the indirect system.
  d **True.**
  e **True.**

10 a **False.** It is largest in a myope.
  b **True.**
  c **True.** That is, the patient's pupil and the observer's pupil are conjugate foci.
  d **False.** The image is laterally and vertically inverted.
  e **True.** Using an aspheric condensing lens, a field of view of 25 degrees may be seen.

11 a **False.**
  b **True.** The eye piece incorporates a $+2\,D$ lens.
  c **True.** A $+13\,D$ lens gives a linear magnification of 5 times, while a $+20\,D$ lens gives a linear magnification of 3 times.
  d **True.** It can be used with a sheet of glass as an image splitter.
  e **True.**

12 a **True.** The higher lens powers have a larger field of view, useful when the patient is not highly cooperative.
  b **True.**
  c **False.** The indirect is preferable. It has a larger field of view and stereopsis can be used to view the detachment.
  d **True.** Although the Volk lens used with the slit lamp is an indirect method which produces high magnification.
  e **False.** The direct ophthalmoscope allows direct viewing of the fundus.

13 a **True.**

   b **True.**

   c **False.** The field of view is smaller in a myope and larger in a hypermetrope.

   d **True.** Hence the advantage of using dilating drops prior to fundal examination.

   e **False.** The field of view enlarges as you approach the patient.

14 a **True.** The image is smaller in hypermetropia and larger in myopia.

   b **True.** A correcting convex lens is required.

   c **False.** See answer (a) – aphakia is an extreme form of hypermetropia.

   d **True.** The correcting lenses are only spherical. This may cause a distorted image in high degrees of astigmatism – in such cases, the patient's spectacles can be left in place.

   e **True.** This is especially useful in examination of patients with retinopathy.

15 a **True.**

   b **False.** When the mirror is at the top, a converging beam is produced with a streak retinoscope, and a parallel beam with a spot retinoscope.

   c **True.** In this model, a "with" movement indicates hypermetropia. The converging beam is very useful for producing a "with" movement in myopia.

   d **False.** The reflex speeds up as neutralisation is reached, and at neutralisation, moves so quickly that its direction cannot be judged.

   e **True.** And when this image is placed in the plane of the retinoscope mirror using lenses, neutralisation is reached.

16 a **True.**

   b **False.** The Placido disc is not used as a keratometer. The two common designs are the one-position instruments, such as the Bausch and Lomb design where doubling can occur in two directions at once, and two-position instruments, such as the Javal–Schiotz, where doubling occurs in one meridian only, and two readings therefore need to be taken (one for each meridian).

   c **False.** The object size is fixed.

   d **False.** In the Javal–Schiotz design, the separation of two objects is varied to alter the doubling and measure the radius.

   e **True.**

17 a **False.** The Placidos disc is flat.
   b **False.** The lens is convex.
   c **False.** It is best positioned behind the subject's head.
   d **False.** It does not give accurate measurements of corneal curvature but instead gives an impression of corneal distortion.
   e **True.**

18 a **True.** Readings are taken by aligning the two images with one another.
   b **True.**
   c **True.**
   d **False.** Keratometers use the first Purkinje reflection.
   e **True.**

19 a **False.** Each step equals 1 D of corneal power.
   b **False.** The image is derived from a convex reflector (the cornea) and is minified and virtual.
   c **False.** The central 3–4 mm of the cornea is measured.
   d **False.** Variable doubling is achieved by altering the distance of a prism (which alters its effective power).
   e **True.**

20 a **False.** Microscopes are focused for near objects.
   b **True.**
   c **True.** This inverts the image so that it is viewed as erect.
   d **False.** Two convex lenses are used.
   e **True.**

21 a **True.**
   b **False.** The image is magnified.
   c **True.**
   d **True.**
   e **True.** It is used to examine and photograph the corneal endothelium.

22 a **False.** The angle of separation is actually 13 degrees.
   b **True.** Transparent structures are difficult to visualise in other ways.
   c **True.** Retro-illumination from the fundus can be used to view lens structures if an opacity is present.
   d **True.**
   e **True.**

23 a **False.** It is a low-powered compound microscope.
   b **True.** Their common axis of rotation also lies in this focal plane.
   c **False.** The distance between the microscope and the subject is reasonably long, allowing manoeuvres like removing a corneal foreign body or use of contact lenses.
   d **True.**
   e **True.** Short wavelength light (blue and green) scatters more than red light. Scatter is necessary to view the vitreous gel.

24 a **False.** The Hruby lens is a concave lens of power $-58\,D$ used to neutralise the cornea and view the fundus.
   b **False.** The fundus is viewed directly.
   c **True.**
   d **False.** Lower lens powers give a decreased field of view and an increased magnification for indirect ophthalmoscopy.
   e **True.** This lens neutralises the corneal power.

25 a **True.** Here the retinal image is found in the pupillary plane.
   b **True.**
   c **True.**
   d **False.** Their central zones may be used to view the posterior pole.
   e **False.** They are convex.

26 a **False.** Indentation tonometers such as the Schiotz measure the force required to indent the cornea – a probe is pushed a certain distance into the cornea. The Goldmann is an applanation tonometer, where an area of cornea is flattened.
   b **True.** This principle measures the force required to produce a fixed area of flattening.
   c **True.** This was chosen by Goldmann, since at this diameter the elastic forces of the cornea (which resist flattening) are balanced by the attractive force of surface tension.
   d **False.** The Perkins relies on the same principle as the Goldmann tonometer.
   e **True.** These produce doubling.

27 a True. This occurs when the area of contact is about 3 mm in diameter.
  b True.
  c True.
  d False.
  e True. When the half circles just overlap, the area of contact is 3.06 mm diameter.

28 a False. Corneal thickness is measured by measuring the amount of doubling required to place one image of the cornea directly behind the other.
  b True.
  c True. A perspex plate is rotated to produce variable doubling.
  d True.
  e True.

29 a True.
  b True.
  c True.
  d False. These are keratometers.
  e False.

30 a True. The potential acuity meter uses a clear window in the cataractous lens to project an acuity chart on the retina. Thus macular function can be assessed even in the presence of a cataract.
  b True.
  c True.
  d True. The small aperture through which the acuity chart is projected gives the image a large depth of field making it resistant to refractive error.
  e True. A clear window is required.

31 a **True.** Scanning laser ophthalmoscopy uses a low light level and infra-red radiation to obtain high resolution images of the retina.

b **True.** A-scan ultrasonography uses a stationary 8 mHz piezo crystal to emit and receive sound waves. By measuring the time delay before a particular signal is received the axial length of the globe is determined.

c **True.** A-scan uses a non-focused parallel beam which emanates from a piezo crystal.

d **True.** B-scan is of particular value in the diagnosis of intra-ocular tumours, retinal detachments, vitreous haemorrhage, and rupture of the globe.

e **False.** Contact and immersion scans are terms relevant to B-scan. The latter is of particular value in scanning the anterior segment.

32 a **True.** The illumination action and observation beams are separate so the instrument is reflex-free.

b **True.** The aerial image is formed between the holed mirror and the ophthalmoscope lens.

c **True.** The fundus camera has a 30 degree field of view and therefore produces excellent photographs of the fundus.

d **True.** The filters are used during fundus fluorescein angiography.

e **True.**

33 a **True.** They are therefore convenient to mechanise and are incorporated in operating microscopes.

b **True.**

c **True.** In compensated systems the image is always at the same position relative to the front element. The compensation is produced either (i) *mechanically*, i.e. by moving the rear element to neutralise the shift in image position or (ii) *optically*, by incorporating additional movable elements.

d **False.** In uncompensated zoom systems, the centre element moves changing the magnification as well as the focus.

e **True.**

113

34 a **True.** In the blue field entoptic test, the patient is asked to look into a blue field. In this situation, the flow of blood in retinal capillaries becomes noticeable. If the patient does not notice this effect, this may indicate non-perfusion of the macular area.

  b **True.** In this test, the patient's acuity is compared with and without a glare source located behind the Snellen chart (on a bright day, a window is an ideal glare source). This test is useful if a patient's acuity appears fairly good, but it is suspected that media opacities are giving rise to symptoms of glare.

  c **False.** Noise charts are contrast sensitivity charts with added visual "noise". Under these circumstances, contrast sensitivity is reduced more by neural damage than by poor optical quality.

  d **True.**

  e **False.** OMDTs are more greatly reduced by retinal damage (such as ARMD) than by reduced optical quality since the task can still be performed in the presence of significant levels of blur.

35 a **False.** The fundus is viewed *directly*.

  b **True.** An inverted, real image of the patient's fundus is viewed.

  c **False.** The lens required in the direct ophthalmoscope is the addition of the examiner's and the patient's refractive errors. For pre-presbyopic examiners and patients, the effect of accommodation is often noticeable (i.e. a relatively myopic correction is required).

  d **False.** The distance at which the lens is held will determine the position of the aerial image.

  e **True.**

Clinical ophthalmology

Questions

1 Benign intracranial hypertension (BIH):

   a Is typically found in young obese females.
   b May result from chronic mastoiditis.
   c Is associated with features of hydrocephalus on a CT scan.
   d Often requires surgical treatment to limit the course of the disease.
   e Is associated with visual disturbances which can be improved with a lumbar peritoneal shunt.

2 The electrooculogram (EOG):

   a Is useful in neonates.
   b Is tested in dark and light adapted states.
   c Produces a trace from which the Arden index can be calculated, dividing the dark trough by the light peak.
   d Is abnormal in asymptomatic patients with Best's disease.
   e Shows an absent light rise in retinitis pigmentosa.

3 Visual evoked potential (VEP)

   The following are true:

   a The signal is generated from the occipital cortex.
   b The VEP is essentially a test of the peripheral retina.
   c Flash VEPs can be used to determine visual acuity in the presence of opaque media.
   d VEPs can be used to detect past episodes of "retrobulbar" neuritis.
   e The VEP assesses the visual system beyond the retinal ganglion cells.

4 Regarding the electroretinogram (ERG):

   a It requires two electrodes to be attached to the medial and lateral canthi.
   b It originates from the photoreceptors and retinal pigment epithelium.
   c Dark adaptation takes 30 minutes and isolates cone responses.
   d Leber's amaurosis causes a purely scotopic response reduction.
   e Retinitis pigmentosa predominantly affects the scotopic response.

5 Albinism

The following are true:

   a Tyrosinase positive oculocutaneous albinism is X-linked recessive.
   b Albinism can be associated with neutrophil abnormalities leading to fatal disease.
   c Ocular albinism carriers show RPE granularity.
   d Tyrosinase negative oculocutaneous albinism is associated with abnormal decussation at the chiasm.
   e Hair bulb incubation is best tested under the age of 5.

6 Blinking may be reduced in:

   a Coma.
   b Drug intoxication.
   c Hyperthyroidism.
   d Progressive supranuclear palsy.
   e Parkinson's disease.

7 Concerning chronic progressive external opthalmoplegia:

   a It is a mitochondrial muscle dystrophy.
   b Muscle biopsy shows ragged red fibres.
   c It is associated with a pigmentary retinopathy.
   d It causes diplopia.
   e It may cause ptosis.

8 Pulsatile proptosis may be caused by:

    a Neurofibromatosis.
    b Caroticocavernous fistulas.
    c Meningoencephalocele.
    d Arteriovenous malformations.
    e Orbital metastases.

9 Caroticocavernous fistula:

    a Most often is the result of trauma.
    b Can cause rubeosis.
    c May resolve spontaneously.
    d Causes a low flow arteriovenous shunt.
    e May be diagnosed by cerebral angiography.

10 Fluorescein angiography

The following are true:

    a Fluorescein normally leaks from the retinal circulation.
    b Time taken for dye to reach the eye from the arm is approximately 9 seconds.
    c The macula appears dark because there is an increased density of RPE cells.
    d The macula appears dark because there is an increased density of melanin.
    e Hypofluorescence may be caused by choroidal ischaemia.

11 Painless partial IIIrd nerve palsies which spare the pupil:

    a Are always ischaemic.
    b Are usually compressive.
    c May be a feature of demyelinating disease.
    d Should have neuro imaging.
    e Are associated with diabetes.

12 Causes of light–near dissociation include:

    a Parinaud's syndrome.
    b Luetic disease.
    c Myotonic dystrophy.
    d Aberrant regeneration of the IIIrd nerve.
    e Myasthenia gravis.

13 Features of type 1 neurofibromatosis include:

    a Lisch nodules.
    b Bilateral acoustic neuromas.
    c Café au lait spots.
    d Astrocytic hamartomas.
    e Prominent corneal nerves.

14 Causes of unilateral temporary visual loss include:

    a Rheumatic fever.
    b Vertebrobasilar disease.
    c Carotid artery disease.
    d Raised intracranial pressure.
    e Retrobulbar neuritis.

15 Colour vision may be tested using:

    a The Ishihara colour chart.
    b The Nagel anomaloscope.
    c The D15 test.
    d The Farnsworth 100 hue test.
    e The Spiza bar.

16 Argyll Robertson pupils:

    a Are bilaterally small and irregular.
    b Exhibit light–near dissociation.
    c Do not accommodate.
    d May be caused by diabetes.
    e May be caused by encephalitis.

17 Causes of a bull's eye maculopathy include:

    a Chloroquine.
    b Batten's disease.
    c Trauma.
    d Cone dystrophy.
    e Benign concentric annular macular dystrophy.

18 Optic disc colobomas:

    a Are caused by incomplete closure of the fetal fissure.
    b Produce non-progressive visual field defects.
    c Are associated with posterior lenticonus.
    d Are associated with microphthalmia.
    e Are associated with corpus callosum agenesis.

19 Horner's syndrome:

    a Causes a complete ptosis.
    b Is associated with facial anhidrosis.
    c May cause heterochromia.
    d May be caused by Hodgkin's disease.
    e Can be confirmed by the hydroxyamphetamine test.

20 Optic disc drusen:

    a Are unilateral in 30% of cases.
    b Exhibit autofluorescence.
    c Are associated with disciforms.
    d Are associated with arterial trifurcation.
    e Are usually acquired.

21 Causes of heterochromia iridis include:

    a Posner–Schlossman syndrome.
    b Congential Horner's syndrome.
    c Waardenberg's syndrome.
    d Parry–Romberg syndrome.
    e Marfan's syndrome.

22 Optic neuritis:

    a Does not occur in children.
    b May be caused by herpes zoster.
    c Is more common in tropical zones.
    d May cause a macular star.
    e Can be associated with paraplegia.

23 Palsies of the IIIrd cranial nerve

The following are true:

    a Unilateral nuclear lesions cause unilateral IIIrd nerve palsy with contralateral superior rectus palsy.
    b Bilateral nuclear lesions cause bilateral IIIrd nerve palsies with sparing of levator palpebrae.
    c Weber's syndrome is the association of contralateral hemitremor with IIIrd nerve palsy.
    d A IIIrd nerve palsy may be caused by herpes zoster.
    e Aberrant regeneration may occur following ischaemic lesions.

24 Causes of optic atrophy include:

    a Heredity.
    b Paget's disease.
    c Mucopolysaccharidoses.
    d Trauma.
    e Diabetic papillopathy.

25 Regarding pituitary tumours:

    a Adenomas are more common in elderly males.
    b They may cause transient unilateral visual loss.
    c They may cause optic atrophy.
    d Surgery has a poor prognosis.
    e A pituitary tumour may present with visual failure alone.

26 Causes of toxic optic neuropathy include:

    a Quinine.
    b Penicillamine.
    c Ethambutol.
    d Fusidic acid.
    e Chloramphenicol.

27 Causes of anterior ischaemic optic neuropathy include:

    a Temporal arteritis.
    b Diabetes mellitus.
    c Carotid artery disease.
    d Systemic hypertension.
    e Systemic hypotension.

28 Regarding trochlear nerve palsies:

    a There is diplopia which is worse on downgaze.
    b There is ipsilateral hypotropia.
    c Abnormal head posture held is chin down with face turn to the ipsilateral side.
    d If congenital, it is always present by age 20.
    e If bilateral, the double Maddox rod test will show more than 10 degrees of torsion.

29 Holmes–Adie pupil:

    a Exhibits sectoral vermiform movements.
    b May have a viral aetiology.
    c Is associated with hyporeflexia in Holmes–Adie syndrome.
    d Always constricts with 0.1% pilocarpine.
    e Exhibits light–near dissociation.

30 Giant cell arteritis

The following are true:

a Small to medium sized arteries are affected.
b The ESR is always high.
c One of the best diagnostic symptoms is jaw claudication.
d It may be associated with proximal limb girdle weakness.
e It may cause anterior segment ischaemia.

31 Acoustic neuromas:

a May cause facial nerve involvement.
b Are found in type I neurofibromatosis.
c May be associated with decreased corneal sensation.
d Are often associated with meningiomas.
e May cause nystagmus.

32 Regarding tuberous sclerosis:

a It may be familial or sporadic.
b There is an association with West's syndrome.
c Ashleaf patches are a feature.
d Café au lait patches are a feature.
e Mulberry tumours are calcified hamartomas.

33 Optic nerve gliomas:

a Are more common in children.
b Are often bilateral.
c Are fast growing.
d Present with proptosis.
e Need early radiotherapy.

122

34 Visual field defects may be caused by:

    a Optic nerve hypoplasia.
    b Myelinated nerve fibres.
    c Optic disc pits.
    d Tilted optic discs.
    e Multiple sclerosis.

35 Parietal lobe lesions

The following are true:

    a Parietal lobe lesions cause a complete homonymous hemianopia.
    b The optokinetic reflex is normal.
    c They are associated with apraxia.
    d There may be sparing of the macula.
    e The most common cause is vascular.

36 Parinaud's syndrome is associated with:

    a Light–near dissociation.
    b Convergence retraction nystagmus.
    c Setting sun sign.
    d Pupil abnormalities.
    e Pinealoma.

37 Causes of pupil abnormalities include:

    a Idiopathic.
    b Trauma.
    c Syringomyelia.
    d Encephalitis.
    e Myotonic dystrophy.

38 Causes of optic disc swelling include:

   a Disc drusen.
   b Benign intracranial hypertension.
   c Ocular hypotony.
   d Lymphoma.
   e Anaemia.

39 Occipital lobe lesions:

   a May have macular sparing.
   b Cause an incongruous hemianopia.
   c Cause abnormal OKN responses.
   d Caused by posterior cerebral artery thrombosis will result in total cortical blindness.
   e Are vascular in origin in 90% of lesions.

40 Diabetic optic neuropathy:

   a Is usually associated with type II diabetes.
   b Is rarely bilateral.
   c Can cause macula oedema.
   d Commonly causes minimal visual disturbance.
   e Needs prompt treatment.

41 A sixth nerve palsy:

   a Causes horizontal diplopia worse at near.
   b Causes a face turn to the opposite side to the lesion.
   c When associated with ipsilateral seventh nerve paresis and contralateral hemiparesis is known as Millard–Gubler syndrome.
   d May be caused by otitis media.
   e Can occur with caroticocavernous fistula.

42 Regarding optic nerve hypoplasia:

    a Causes include maternal alcoholism.
    b It may cause pupil abnormalities.
    c Vision is normal.
    d Associations include aniridia.
    e Associations include De Morsier's syndrome.

43 The following are associated with Parkinson's disease:

    a Reduced saccades.
    b Seborrhoeic blepharitis.
    c Reduced blinking.
    d Progressive gaze palsy.
    e Pill rolling tremor.

44 Multiple sclerosis causes:

    a Retrobulbar neuritis.
    b Red desaturation.
    c Uhthoff's phenomenon.
    d Pulfrich's phenomenon.
    e One and a half syndrome.

45 Ocular motility

The field of binocular single vision (BSV):

    a Is useful in assessing patients with diplopia.
    b Is plotted using a perimeter.
    c Depicts the areas of diplopia.
    d Uses a red target for fixation.
    e Requires presbyopic patients to wear reading glasses in order to perform this test.

46 Regarding binocular single vision (BSV):

    a The field of BSV is narrow and relatively central in a blow-out fracture.

    b The smaller the field of BSV the greater the limitation of ocular movement.

    c The size of the field of BSV is influenced by the amplitude of fusion.

    d The field of BSV is of little value in a patient with a normal Hess chart.

    e The field of BSV can be normal in a patient with an abnormal Hess chart.

47 The forced duction test:

    a Is used to assess active movement of the globe.

    b Requires local anaesthesia.

    c Can be positive in neurogenic palsies.

    d Will be positive in restrictive causes of under-acting extraocular muscles.

    e Must ideally be performed at the start of any strabismus surgery.

48 Myogenic palsies include:

    a Myasthenia gravis.

    b Ocular myositis.

    c Eaton–Lambert–Rooke syndrome.

    d Chronic progressive external ophthalmoplegia.

    e Brown's syndrome.

49 Regarding myasthenia gravis:

    a Any age group can be affected.

    b It is usually transient in neonates.

    c Ocular muscles are often the first to be involved.

    d It is due to a deficiency of acetyl choline.

    e Horizontal diplopia is the classic presentation.

50 Myasthenia gravis

The following are true:

a The Tensilon test is used to diagnose myasthenia.
b The diplopia is variable and improves with effort.
c The Tensilon test must be carried out with ready access to resuscitation facilities.
d Edrophonium is an anticholinergic drug.
e A negative Tensilon test rules out myasthenia.

51 Ocular myasthenia may be managed by:

a Prisms.
b Surgery.
c Botulinum toxin.
d Ptosis props.
e Immunosuppressants.

52 Dysthyroid eye disease

The following are true:

a Superior rectus is the muscle most commonly affected.
b Superior rectus involvement causes limitation of upgaze.
c Muscle enlargement can be seen on CT scan.
d Forced duction test may be positive.
e Differential intra-ocular pressure gives some indication of the direction of maximum restriction.

53 Thyroid ophthalmopathy may be managed by:

a Steroids.
b Immunosuppressants.
c Prisms.
d Botulinum toxin.
e Surgery.

54 Amblyopia

The following are true:

a Amblyopia is defined as defective visual acuity in one or both eyes persisting after correction of the refractive error.
b It can be due to a squint.
c Strabismic amblyopia is more common with exotropia.
d A ptosis can cause amblyopia.
e It can be reversed in an adult with correction of the refractive error.

55 The following are true:

a Panum's area is essential for BSV.
b Stimulation of disparate retinal elements within Panum's area allows fusion of images.
c A microtropia is detected with a 4 D prism.
d Patients with microtropia have normal BSV.
e A patient with microtropia will usually see 4 lights with the Worth's four-lights test.

56 The following are true:

a "V" pattern is usually due to underaction of the superior rectus muscle.
b "A" pattern is caused by underaction of the inferior rectus.
c In a "V" pattern the esodeviation increases on downgaze.
d In an "A" pattern the exodeviation increases on upgaze.
e "V" pattern is seen in association with Brown's syndrome.

57 Duane's syndrome

The following are true:

a Duane's syndrome is caused by contraction of the horizontal recti.
b It is seen in Goldenhar's syndrome.
c It may follow excessive lateral rectus resection.
d It can be due to aplasia of the IVth nerve nucleus.
e There is narrowing of the palpebral fissure on abduction.

128

58 Regarding Brown's syndrome:

    a Congenital cases improve with time.
    b The "bridle" phenomenon is a classic feature.
    c Forced duction testing is usually positive.
    d A click may be heard.
    e It is bilateral in 30% of cases.

59 The following are true:

    a Surgery is necessary in all cases of orbital floor fractures.
    b Diplopia can be a late complication of retinal detachment surgery.
    c Diplopia secondary to mechanical restriction by an explant is successfully treated by removing the explant.
    d Orbital tumours can cause diplopia.
    e Orbital myositis can cause diplopia.

60 Regarding Brown's syndrome:

    a Limitation of adduction is the main sign.
    b Overaction of the inferior oblique is present.
    c It can be secondary to a short tendon sheath.
    d It can be secondary to a short superior oblique tendon.
    e Swelling of the tendon can be a cause.

61 Ptosis

The following are true:

    a Ptosis in the Marcus Gunn syndrome is due to misdirection of the facial nerve.
    b Aponeurotic ptosis may follow ocular surgery.
    c The blepharophimosis syndrome is an example of mechanical ptosis.
    d Congenital ptosis may be associated with astigmatism.
    e Underaction of the superior rectus may be seen in congenital ptosis.

62 The following are true:

a Myotonic dystrophy is a cause of ptosis.
b Ocular myopathy is a cause of ptosis.
c Blepharophimosis is an autosomal recessive trait.
d Amblyopia is seen in 50% of patients with the blepharophimosis syndrome.
e Hypertelorism is a feature of the blepharophimosis syndrome.

63 Fundus fluorescein angiography (FFA)

The following are true:

a Fluorescein can cross the inner blood–retinal barrier.
b Up to 85% of fluorescein in the circulation is bound to proteins.
c Fluorescein is mainly excreted by the kidneys.
d Two filters are used in FFA.
e The excitation peak of fluorescein is at 530 nm.

64 Regarding fluorescein angiogram (FFA):

a The choroidal circulation is best studied by fluorescein angiography.
b Hypofluorescence is seen in severe myopia.
c In papilloedema, the optic disc may show leakage in the arterial phase.
d Adverse reactions to intravenous fluorescein include bronchospasm and anaphylactic shock.
e Late staining of the optic disc is suggestive of papilloedema.

65 CT scan

The following are true:

a A CT scan uses thin X-ray beams.
b The location of a space occupying orbital lesion can be determined with a CT scan.
c CT scan is useful to differentiate a benign tumour from a malignant one.
d Bone is well defined on a CT scan.
e The muscle tendon is normal in dysthyroid ophthalmopathy on a CT scan.

66 CT scan shows:

    a Fusiform enlargement of the muscle in myositis.

    b Fusiform enlargement of the optic nerve in optic nerve sheath meningioma.

    c Calcification of the optic nerve in optic nerve sheath meningioma.

    d Plaques of demyelination in most patients with multiple sclerosis.

    e Bony excavation of the lacrimal gland fossa in a benign lacrimal gland tumour.

67 Magnetic resonance imaging (MRI):

    a MRI uses an electromagnetic pulse.

    b The vitreous is dark on T_2 weighted images.

    c Gadolinium is used as a contrast.

    d Orbital fat is hyperintense on T_1 weighted images.

    e MRI is an unsuitable form of investigation for patients with claustrophobia.

68 Regarding slit lamp examination:

    a Direct illumination is used to detect gross abnormalities.

    b A cross section of the cornea is visualised with direct illumination.

    c The location and depth of a lesion in the cornea can be assessed by direct illumination.

    d The slit beam is directed to illuminate the cornea from behind in scleral scatter.

    e Guttata are best seen by retro-illumination.

69 The following are true:

    a The Caldwell view on skull X-rays is useful to detect orbital floor fractures.

    b The patient's chin is slightly elevated for a Waters' view.

    c Orbital lesions are seen in a Caldwell view.

    d The "tear drop" sign is best seen in a Waters' view.

    e The superior orbital fissure can be identified in a Caldwell view.

70 Indocyanine green (ICG):

    a Has low fluorescence as compared to fluorescein.
    b Does not escape from the choriocapillaris.
    c Can be used in individuals allergic to iodine.
    d Absorbs and reflects in the ultra-violet portion of the spectrum.
    e Is useful in defining choroidal new vessels.

71 Hess charts

The following are true:

    a The smaller field indicates the affected eye.
    b The Hess chart shows the position of the fixing eye in all positions of gaze.
    c A difference in the size of the fields usually indicates a recent onset paresis.
    d "A" and "V" patterns can be seen on a Hess chart.
    e No deviation in the primary position may be seen in a mechanical lesion.

72 The following are true:

    a On a Hess chart, a mechanical lesion shows significant muscle sequelae.
    b Neurogenic palsies have compressed fields on a Hess chart.
    c Deviation in primary position is seen in neurogenic palsies.
    d In longstanding neurogenic palsies, some degree of comitance is often seen.
    e Sloping fields are seen in neurogenic palsies.

73 Exophthalmometry

The following are true:

    a Exophthalmometry measures the degree of proptosis.
    b Measurements are taken with the exophthalmometer resting on the supra-orbital ridge.
    c A difference of 2 mm between the two eyes is suspicious.
    d Exophthalmometry measures the distance between the apex of the cornea and the supra-orbital ridge.
    e A reading of 18 mm suggests proptosis.

74 Regarding infantile esotropia:

    a A large angle esotropia is seen.
    b Cross fixation is seen.
    c It is usually associated with high hypermetropia.
    d Inferior oblique overaction, if present, usually remains unilateral.
    e Surgery can be delayed until the child goes to school.

75 The following are true:

    a A high AC/A ratio is seen in non-refractive accommodative esotropia.
    b Fully accommodative esotropia is seen with high refractive errors.
    c Congenital exotropias are invariably present at birth.
    d Congenital esotropias are invariably present at birth.
    e Spectacle correction in a myope may control all or part of an exodeviation.

76 The following are true:

    a Intermittent exotropia becomes noticeable when the child is day-dreaming.
    b Intermittent exotropias may become constant as the child grows older.
    c Sensory deprivation which occurs before the age of 5 can produce an esodeviation.
    d Dissociated vertical deviation (DVD) is characteristically seen in an accommodative esotropia.
    e Bifocals are used in the management of accommodative esotropia with a high AC/A ratio.

Clinical ophthalmology

Answers

1 **a** **True.**
  b **True.** This may cause spread of inflammation to the sigmoid and lateral sinuses causing venous sinus thrombosis.
  c **False.** BIH causes parenchymal swelling and hence the ventricles are often smaller than usual.
  d **False.** BIH is usually a self-limiting disease and most cases respond to simple conservative treatment. Usual treatment measures include weight loss and cessation of any predisposing medication, e.g. the oral contraceptive pill, tetracyclines, diuretics, acetazolamide (reduces CSF production).
  e **True.** This is highly effective in reversing symptoms and improving papilloedema.

2 **a** **False.** It needs the patient to look from side to side and hence is inappropriate for the very young.
  b **True.**
  c **False.** It is the light peak divided by the dark trough. Its value is normally 185%.
  d **True.**
  e **True.** Widespread retinal pigment epithelial damage causes EOG abnormalities.

3 **a** **True.**
  b **False.** It principally tests macular function.
  c **False.** They are only able to test whether light is perceived. Pattern VEPs may be used to test acuity.
  d **True.** Amplitude is normal but latency is reduced in healed optic neuritis.
  e **True.**

4 a **False.** One electrode is placed on the cornea while the other is placed on the forehead.
  b **False.** It originates from the photoreceptors and bipolar cells.
  c **False.** It isolates rod responses.
  d **False.** Both photopic and scotopic responses are severely reduced.
  e **True.** It causes nyctalopia.

5 a **False.** Oculocutaneous albinism is autosomal recessive.
  b **True.** The Chediak–Higashi syndrome involves recurrent infections and fatal disease with mild albinism.
  c **True.** They may also have iris transillumination.
  d **True.** 90% of fibres decussate at the chiasm.
  e **False.** It is best tested after 4 years of age.

6 a **True.** Reduced conscious level is associated with reduced blinking.
  b **True.** For example, alcohol.
  c **False.** Hypothyroidism causes decreased blinking.
  d **True.**
  e **True.**

7 a **True.**
  b **True.**
  c **True.**
  d **False.** As the ophthalmoplegia is symmetrical, patients do not get diplopia.
  e **True.**

8 a **True.**
  b **True.**
  c **True.**
  d **True.**
  e **False.**

9 a **True.**
   b **True.**
   c **True.** 5% spontaneously resolve, 50% result in loss of vision.
   d **True.** Flow may be high or low flow.
   e **True.**

10 a **False.** It leaks from the choroidal circulation but normally stays intravascular in the retina.
   b **True.**
   c **True.**
   d **True.**
   e **True.** Other causes include masking, retinal ischaemia, and atrophy of vascular tissue, e.g. in myopia.

11 a **False.** Occasionally aneurysms may present in this way.
   b **False.** They are commonly ischaemic.
   c **True.**
   d **True.** To exclude a compressive lesion.
   e **True.**

12 a **True.**
   b **True.**
   c **True.**
   d **True.**
   e **False.**

13 a **True.**
   b **False.** These are found in type II.
   c **True.**
   d **True.** Found in approximately 30% of cases.
   e **True.**

14 a **True.**
   b **False.**
   c **True.**
   d **True.**
   e **True.**

15 a **True.**
  b **True.**
  c **True.**
  d **True.**
  e **False.**

16 a **True.**
  b **True.**
  c **False.** They accommodate but do not respond to the direct light test.
  d **True.**
  e **True.**

17 a **True.**
  b **True.**
  c **False.**
  d **True.**
  e **True.**

18 a **True.**
  b **True.**
  c **True.** They are also associated with posterior embryotoxon and non-rhegmatogenous retinal detachment.
  d **True.**
  e **True.** Other systemic abnormalities associated include Meckel–Gruber, sphenoidal encephalocele, and the CHARGE syndrome.

19 a **False.** It causes a mild (2 mm) ptosis.
  b **True.** If the lesion is pre-ganglionic facial anhydrosis may occur.
  c **True.** Longstanding Horner's syndrome causes heterochromia.
  d **True.** Other lesions of the cervical sympathetic chain include a carotid aneurysm or carotid body tumour.
  e **False.** The cocaine test is used to confirm a Horner's syndrome of any order, whereas the hydroxyamphetamine test is used to differentiate pre-ganglionic from post-ganglionic Horner's syndrome.

137

20 a **True.**
   b **True.**
   c **True.** They may also be associated with vitreous haemorrhage, angioid streaks, and retinitis pigmentosa.
   d **True.**
   e **False.** They are usually congenital and often familial.

21 a **True.**
   b **True.**
   c **True.** This syndrome includes congenital deafness, telecanthus, and a white forelock as its other features.
   d **True.** Here heterochromia is associated with Horner's syndrome, oculomotor palsies, facial hemiatrophy, and nystagmus.
   e **False.**

22 a **False.** Devic's disease affects children and young adults.
   b **True.** Other viral causes include Epstein–Barr.
   c **False.** It is more common in temperate zones.
   d **True.**
   e **True.** In neuromyelitis optica (Devic's disease), viral encephalitis causes a rapid onset of bilateral visual loss with paraplegia.

23 a **True.**
   b **True.**
   c **False.** This is Benedict's syndrome. Weber's is a lesion of the cerebral peduncle causing an associated contralateral hemiparesis.
   d **True.** Other causes include diabetes, atherosclerosis, vasculitis, and migraine.
   e **False.** Aberrant regeneration will only occur secondary to IIIrd nerve paresis caused by tumour or trauma. Primary aberrant regeneration with no preceding acute IIIrd nerve palsy is indicative of an intracavernous lesion.

24 a **True.** These include Leber's hereditary optic neuropathy and congenital syphilis.
   b **True.** Bony overgrowth causes compressive atrophy.
   c **True.**
   d **True.**
   e **False.** Recovery from this condition usually occurs within six months.

25 a **False.** Adenomas have no sex predilection and usually occur in middle aged adults.
  b **True.**
  c **True.**
  d **False.** Trans-sphenoidal hypophysectomy has a good success rate.
  e **True.** Non-secreting adenomas may initially present with visual symptoms alone.

26 a **True.**
  b **True.**
  c **True.**
  d **False.**
  e **True.** This occurs more frequently in children.

27 a **True.**
  b **True.**
  c **True.**
  d **True.**
  e **True.**

28 a **True.**
  b **False.** These palsies cause ipsilateral hypertropia.
  c **False.** Face turn is to the opposite side.
  d **False.** They may present over the age of 40 when decompensation occurs.
  e **True.**

29 a **True.**
  b **True.**
  c **True.**
  d **False.** An acute Adie's pupil has not had time to develop hypersensitivity.
  e **True.**

30 a **False.** It affects large to medium sized arteries.
  b **False.** It is normal in approximately 30% of cases.
  c **True.**
  d **True.** Polymyalgia rheumatica is often associated.
  e **True.** Other ocular side effects include anterior ischaemic optic neuropathy, oculomotor nerve palsies, and cortical blindness.

31 a **True.**
  b **False.** Type II.
  c **True.**
  d **True.**
  e **True.** Cerebellar involvement causes nystagmus.

32 a **True.** It is autosomal dominant, with 50% being new mutations.
  b **True.** This comprises mental handicap and epilepsy.
  c **True.** These are hypopigmented spots, more visible under ultraviolet light.
  d **True.**
  e **True.**

33 a **True.** More than three-quarters occur in children.
  b **False.**
  c **False.** They are slow growing.
  d **False.** They usually present with visual loss.
  e **False.** Usually treatment is conservative.

34 a **True.**
  b **True.**
  c **True.**
  d **True.**
  e **True.**

35 a **True.**
  b **False.** OKN is reduced towards the side of the lesion.
  c **True.**
  d **False.** This occurs in occipital lobe lesions.
  e **False.** The most common causes are tumours – primary and secondary.

36 a   True.
  b   True.
  c   True.
  d   True. Both pupils are semi-dilated.
  e   True. Other causes include demyelinating diseases and teratoma.

37 a   True. 20% of normals have essential anisocoria.
  b   True. Mydriasis occurs.
  c   True. Cervical cord lesions may cause a Horner's syndrome.
  d   True. This may cause Argyll Robertson pupils.
  e   True. Light–near dissociation occurs in myotonic dystrophy.

38 a   False. Disc drusen cause pseudopapilloedema.
  b   True.
  c   True.
  d   True.
  e   True.

39 a   True.
  b   False. The hemianopia is congruous.
  c   False. Parietal lobe lesions cause an abnormal OKN.
  d   False. There is some overlap with the middle cerebral artery preserving some vision.
  e   True.

40 a   False. It is associated with type I and usually occurs in the second to third decades.
  b   False. 75% of cases are bilateral.
  c   True.
  d   False.
  e   False. Spontaneous recovery usually occurs within six months.

41 a   False. Diplopia is worse in the distance.
  b   False. Face turn is towards the lesion.
  c   True. The lesion will be in the brain stem.
  d   True. This is Gradenigo's syndrome.
  e   True.

42 a **True.**
   b **True.** Unilateral hypoplasia causes a relative afferent pupillary defect.
   c **False.** Vision is usually poor.
   d **True.**
   e **True.**

43 a **True.**
   b **True.**
   c **True.**
   d **False.** This occurs in Steele–Richardson syndrome.
   e **True.**

44 a **True.**
   b **True.**
   c **True.** This is sudden worsening of visual symptoms on exercise or increased temperature.
   d **True.**
   e **True.** This lesion affects the medial longitudinal fasciculus and horizontal gaze centre.

45 a **True.** This test is used in patients with binocular diplopia to assess the area of binocular single vision.
   b **True.**
   c **True.** The areas of diplopia and binocular single vision can be plotted.
   d **False.** A 2 degree white target is used. When the patient cannot see this target, a spotlight is used.
   e **True.** This should be avoided if possible.

46 a True. This is seen in mechanically caused restriction of movement in opposing directions. The field is usually displaced away from the direction of maximum limitation.

b True.

c True. If the amplitude is good the field will be enlarged, especially in neurogenic palsies.

d False. The field of BSV covers a much larger area than the Hess chart. It can therefore be useful in patients with troublesome diplopia but normal Hess charts.

e True. With good fusion amplitude, troublesome diplopia can be overcome and a normal field of BSV attained even in the presence of an obviously displaced Hess chart.

47 a False. The passive movement of the globe is assessed with this test.

b True. Although topical anaesthesia is often used, the patient may still experience discomfort. General anaesthetics, with the exception of succinyl choline which can produce sustained muscle contraction, are preferred.

c True. Neurogenic palsies can have a restrictive element.

d True.

e True.

48 a True. Myogenic palsy is a weakness of muscle movement due to a primary problem in the muscle itself and is distinct from neurogenic palsies and mechanical restrictions. Myasthenia gravis is an autoimmune disease characterised by premature muscle fatigue.

b True. Myositis is an inflammation of the muscles.

c True. This is an acquired weakness of muscles often associated with a systemic malignancy.

d True. CPEO is an inherited degeneration of muscle fibres.

e False. This is a mechanical restriction.

49 a **True.** It may affect the adult as well as the paediatric patient.

  b **True.** Neonatal myasthenia is a self-limiting condition resolving within 4–6 weeks and is seen in babies born to myasthenic mothers.

  c **True.** Diplopia and ptosis are often the presenting symptoms.

  d **False.** Myasthenia gravis is due to depletion of acetyl choline receptors rather than acetyl choline itself.

  e **False.** Vertical diplopia is the classic presentation although any muscle can be involved.

50 a **True.**

  b **False.** The diplopia worsens with fatigue in myasthenia, but may improve in Eaton–Lambert–Rooke syndrome.

  c **True.** Bradycardia and cardiac arrest are among the serious adverse reactions associated with this test.

  d **False.** It is an anticholinesterase and is therefore a cholinergic drug.

  e **False.** Some myasthenics do not respond to anticholinesterase and may therefore show a negative response. In chronically affected muscles a negative response is sometimes seen.

51 a **True.** Prisms can be used to obtain binocular single vision, but may not help when the deviation is large and variable.

  b **True.** Surgery may only be tried when the condition has stabilised.

  c **False.** Botulinum is used to weaken the action of the muscle and cannot be used to treat myasthenia.

  d **True.** Props are mounted on spectacle frames or on contact lenses.

  e **True.** Azathioprine and systemic steroids have been used.

52 a **False.** Inferior rectus followed by the medial rectus are the more commonly involved muscles.

  b **False.** Superior rectus involvement causes limitation of downgaze, the restriction being opposite to the muscle's action.

  c **True.**

  d **True.**

  e **True.** The IOP is measured in primary gaze, upgaze, dextroversion and laevoversion. A rise of 6 mm of IOP indicates mechanical restriction.

53 a **True.** Steroids are used in the presence of compressive optic neuropathy.

  b **True.** Azathioprine may be used with or instead of steroids.

  c **True.** Prisms are useful to restore some useful field of single vision.

  d **True.**

  e **True.** Surgery must however be attempted only when the medical condition and the strabismus have been stable.

54 a **False.** The definition is defective visual acuity in one or both eyes persisting after correction of the refractive error *and* any ocular pathology, e.g. media opacities, ptosis etc.

  b **True.**

  c **False.** It is more common with esotropia. Exotropia tends to be intermittent during childhood, allowing the eye to gain its maximum visual potential.

  d **True.** A ptosis which covers or obstructs the visual axis can produce a stimulus deprivation amblyopia.

  e **False.** The critical period for visual development is from birth to about 8 years, after which correction of amblyopia is not possible.

55 a **True.** Panum's fusional area is an imaginary area that surrounds the horopter in which objects are seen singly. Objects in front of or behind it are seen as double.

  b **True.**

  c **False.** A microtropia, if suspected on a cover test, is assessed for a suppression scotoma with a 4 D prism test. A microesotropia is tested with a base out 4 D prism, whereas a microexotropia is tested with a base in 4 dioptre prism.

  d **False.** In the presence of a microtropia, stereoacuity is usually worse than 40 seconds of arc.

  e **True.** Unless a large heterophoria or intermittent strabismus becomes decompensated.

56 a **True.** "V" pattern is usually due to underaction of the superior oblique or superior rectus.

 b **True.** It can also be caused by underaction of the inferior oblique.

 c **True.**

 d **False.** The exodeviation increases on downgaze in an "A" pattern, whereas the esodeviation increases on upgaze.

 e **True.** The "V" pattern is seen as a divergence on upgaze.

57 a **True.**

 b **True.** Other associations include Klippel–Feil syndrome and deafness.

 c **True.** It can also occur following orbital inflammation.

 d **False.** It is thought to be due to aplasia of the VIth nerve nucleus in some cases.

 e **False.** The palpebral fissure narrows on adduction and the globe retracts into the orbit due to the co-contraction of the horizontal recti.

58 a **False.** Congenital cases are constant whereas the acquired cases are intermittent and resolve with time.

 b **False.** The "Bridle" or "Leash" phenomenon is seen with Duane's syndrome as the tight lateral rectus slips over or under the globe.

 c **True.** It is best elicited when attempting to elevate the eye from the adducted position.

 d **True.** A "click" is sometimes heard as the superior oblique slips through the trochlear.

 e **False.** It is bilateral in about 10% of cases.

59 a **False.** Surgery is indicated only in the presence of (i) persistent diplopia, (ii) incarceration of soft tissue which is unlikely to regress, or (iii) enophthalmos exceeding 3 mm.

 b **True.** Mechanical restriction of the muscle overlying the explant used in retinal detachment surgery or damage to the muscle's nerve supply or a tight encircling band can cause diplopia.

 c **False.** Surgical removal of the explant often does not solve the problem of diplopia as there is additional fibrosis in most cases.

 d **True.**

 e **True.**

60 a False. Limitation of elevation in adduction is the chief sign.
  b True. In some cases the ipsilateral inferior oblique may overact resulting in an upshoot when the eye is adducted beyond the midline.
  c True.
  d True. As is seen following plication of the superior oblique tendon in the surgical treatment of IVth nerve palsy.
  e True. A nodule or swelling on the superior oblique tendon prevents its free passage through the trochlear. A "click" can be heard or felt on attempted elevation in abduction.

61 a False. It is thought to be due to an anomalous innervation of the levator palpebrae superioris by fibres from the Vth nerve.
  b True. Following eye surgery, for example surgery for cataract, glaucoma, retinal detachment etc., manipulation of the superior rectus–levator complex can disinsert the levator aponeurosis leading to an aponeurotic ptosis.
  c False. Blepharophimosis is an example of myogenic ptosis.
  d True. Anisometropia and astigmatism frequently accompany congenital ptosis and are often responsible for the amblyopia seen in these patients.
  e True. This is because of the close embryological relationship between the superior rectus and the levator.

62 a True.
  b True.
  c False. It is an autosomal dominant tract.
  d True.
  e False. Telecanthus, i.e. lateral displacement of the medial canthus, is a feature of the blepharophimosis syndrome. Other features include ptosis, epicanthus inversus, ectropion, and hypoplasia of the superior orbital rims.

63 a False. The tight junctions of the retinal capillary endothelium do not allow the fluorescein molecule to cross this barrier.

  b True.

  c True. This is noticed as an orange discoloration of the urine within 24 hours of the intravenous injection.

  d True. The blue excitation filter and the yellow–green barrier filter are the main filters used in the FFA. When light from the camera passes through the former, blue light emerges and excites the fluorescein molecule in the retinal circulation. The barrier filter ensures that only yellow–green light leaves the eye and is recorded as the fluorescence seen by the observer.

  e False. The excitation peak is 490 nm and the emission peak is 530 nm.

64 a False. The choroidal circulation is poorly discerned with FFA because of the rapid leakage of the fluorescein molecules from the choriocapillaris and because of the blockage by melanin in the RPE. This phase is better studied with indocyanine green (ICG).

  b True. Hypofluorescence in myopia is due to loss of vascular tissue.

  c False. The leakage is in the late venous phase.

  d True. Others include nausea, vomiting, syncope, skin rashes, and laryngeal oedema.

  e False. This is a normal finding.

65 a True. Tissue density values are computed with the help of thin X-ray beams and detailed cross-sectional images formed.

  b True.

  c False. The CT scan cannot distinguish different pathological soft tissue masses which are radiologically isodense.

  d True. In this respect it is superior to MRI.

  e True. This is in contrast to orbital pseudotumour where both the tendon and the belly of the muscle are seen to be involved on CT scan.

66 a **True.**
   b **False.** Fusiform enlargement of the optic nerve is seen in optic nerve glioma.
   c **True.** Calcification and tubular thickening of the optic nerve is seen.
   d **False.** Demyelinating plaques are best seen on MRI.
   e **True.** This excavation is not associated with bone destruction which is seen in a malignant tumour.

67 a **True.** Hydrogen nuclei in the tissues are re-arranged when exposed to this pulse and generate an electromagnetic echo. These echo signals are analysed and computed as a cross-sectional image.
   b **False.** The vitreous is bright on T_2 weighted images
   c **True.**
   d **True.** Fat appears bright (hyperintense) on T_1 weighted images.
   e **True.**

68 a **True.** The slit beam is directed obliquely so that a quadrilateral cross-section of the cornea is visualised.
   b **True.**
   c **True.**
   d **False.** Light falling on the limbus is transmitted within the cornea by total internal reflection and this is the underlying principle in scleral scatter. It is used to detect corneal oedema and subtle opacities.
   e **True.** Retro-illumination, as the name suggests, uses the reflection of light from the iris to illuminate the cornea from behind.

69 a **False.** The Waters' view is preferred in suspected orbital floor fractures.
   b **True.**
   c **True.**
   d **True.** The "tear drop" sign is seen when soft tissue is entrapped in a fracture of the orbital floor and is best seen in a Waters' view.
   e **True.**

149

70 a True. It has a fluorescence of only 4% compared to fluorescein.

  b True. It is highly protein bound and therefore does not escape from the choriocapillaris.

  c False. For intravenous use, ICG is dissolved in an aqueous solvent which contains sodium iodide and cannot be used in patients allergic to iodine.

  d False. It absorbs at 805 nm and reflects at 835 nm which lie in the infra-red range.

  e True. With ICG, the choroid can be visualised even through haemorrhage or pigment deposits in the RPE or retina.

71 a True.

  b False. Hess charts show the position of the non-fixing eye in all positions of gaze when the other eye is fixing.

  c True. A difference in size of the fields of the two eyes indicates incomitance and is usually suggestive of a recent onset paresis.

  d True. "A" or "V" patterns can be seen by sloping sides to the fields on Hess charts.

  e True.

72 a False. In contrast to a neurogenic palsy, a mechanical lesion produces limited muscle sequelae.

  b False. Compressed fields suggest a mechanical cause.

  c True. The deviation in primary position also reflects the extent of the defect.

  d True. Muscle sequelae follow with time in neurogenic palsies producing comitance. Therefore, in a longstanding neurogenic palsy, it may be difficult to discern the primary lesion on a Hess chart.

  e True.

73 a True.

  b False. The exophthalmometer is held so that the two ends rest on the bone at the lateral canthus.

  c True. Any reading above 21 mm or a difference of 2 mm is abnormal.

  d False. The distance between the corneal apex and the lateral orbital rim is measured.

  e False. See answer (c).

74 a **True.** The deviation is fairly large (>30 D) and constant.

  b **True.** The child uses his right eye to fix in left gaze and the left to fix in right gaze.

  c **False.** The refractive error is usually normal for the child's eye.

  d **False.** Even if the inferior oblique overaction is unilateral initially, it frequently becomes bilateral.

  e **False.** The eyes should ideally be aligned by two years so that visual alignment is achieved and the child develops peripheral fusion and some useful binocular single vision.

75 a **True.** This type shows no significant refractive error with little or no deviation for distance, but a significant esodeviation for near best elicited with an accommodative target.

  b **True.** A normal AC/A ratio and high hypermetropia are seen.

  c **True.** Congenital exotropias are also associated with a high incidence of neurological abnormalities.

  d **False.** Most congenital esotropias are not seen at birth but develop within the first six months of life.

  e **True.** It is therefore important to refract the patient with strabismus. Myopic corrections are usually given in full to a patient with exotropia, while hypermetropia if present is under-corrected.

76 a **True.** Bright light, ill health, and day-dreaming can unmask an intermittent exotropia.

  b **True.**

  c **True.** If this occurs after the age of 5 years, an exotropia may result.

  d **False.** It is classically seen in infantile esotropia as an updrift with excyclodeviation of the eye under cover.

  e **True.**

Part Two

OSCE Questions

Optics

Question 1

These are focimeter readings. What is the power of these lenses?

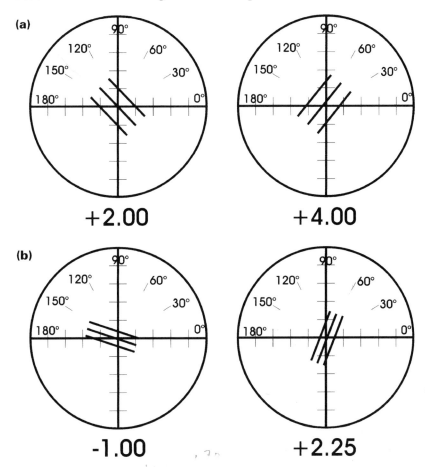

(a)

+2.00

+4.00

(b)

-1.00

+2.25

Answer 1

a   +2.00 DS / +2.00 DC axis 45.
b   −1.00 DS / +3.25 DC axis 80.

The image of the target is seen as a ring of dots when a spherical lens is tested. When reading an astigmatic lens, the target is focused separately for the two principal meridians, seen as line foci. Adjust the focimeter until one set of line foci is sharply in focus; note this reading. Further adjust until a second set of line foci come into focus 90 degrees from the first; note this reading and the axis of the second reading, by reading off the graticule. The first reading gives the spherical power of the lens; the cylindrical power is the algebraic subtraction of the first reading from the second, the axis of the cylinder corresponds to the axis of the second reading.

a   +2.00
    +4.00 − +2.00 = +2.00 axis 45
    +2.00 DS / +2.00 DC axis 45
b   −1.00
    +2.25 − −1.00 = +3.25 axis 80
    −1.00 DS / +3.25 DC axis 80

Question 2

a   By what principle does the focimeter work?
b   Why is it important to note which surface of the lens is placed against the holder of the focimeter?
c   How can the focimeter be used to determine the amount of prism at any given point in a spectacle lens?

Answer 2

a   The focimeter operates on the optometer principle. It consists of a collimator and telescope. Movement of a target allows vergence of light emerging from the collimating lens to be varied; the target is moved until a focused image of it is viewed through the telescope. The distance through which the target is moved is directly related to the dioptric power of the lens under test.
b   The focimeter measures vertex power of a lens, therefore it is important to mount the glasses with the back surface against the holder so that the *back* vertex power is measured.

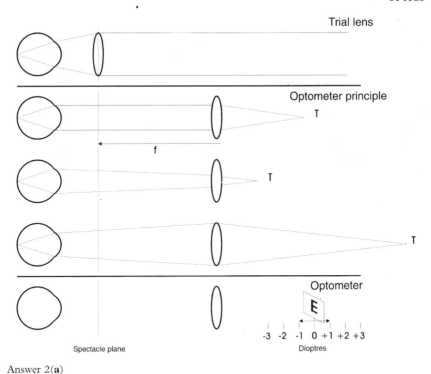

Trial lens

Optometer principle

T

f

T

T

Optometer

E

-3 -2 -1 0 +1 +2 +3

Dioptres

Spectacle plane

Answer 2(**a**)

c A spectacle lens may have a prismatic effect either because prism is incorporated into it or because it has been decentred. To measure prism that is incorporated into a lens, the focimeter image of the focused target will be displaced from the centre of the graticule, the cross-lines of the graticule are calibrated in intervals of one prism dioptre, the direction of displacement from the centre indicates the prism *base*.

The prismatic effect of a decentred lens can be calculated by first using the focimeter to mark the optical centre then placing the spectacles on the patient and measuring the distance between the centre of the patient's pupil and the marked optical centre. Using the Prentice equation:

prismatic power $P = F \times D$

P = prismatic power in prism dioptres
F = lens power in dioptres
D = decentration in centimetres

157

Question 3

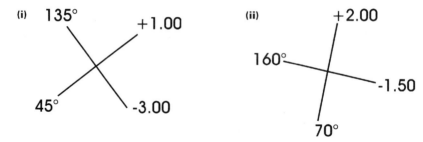

Express these power cross diagrams in:
a   plus cylinder form
b   minus cylinder form

Answer 3

a   (i) $-3.00\,\text{DS}\,/\,+4.00\,\text{DC}$ axis 135   (ii) $-1.50\,\text{DS}\,/\,+3.50\,\text{DC}$ axis 160
b   (i) $+1.00\,\text{DS}\,/\,-4.00\,\text{DC}$ axis 45   (ii) $+2.00\,\text{DS}\,/\,-3.50\,\text{DC}$ axis 70

Question 4

$-2.00\,\text{DS}\,/\,+4.00\,\text{DC}$ axis 100

a   During subjective refraction the cylinder in this prescription is reduced by 50% and the axis is rotated to 90 degrees. What is the resultant prescription if the spherical equivalent is to be kept constant?
b   What is the spherical equivalent?

Answer 4

a $-1.00\,\text{DS}\,/\,+2.00\,\text{DC}$ axis 90
   Add half as much sphere algebraically as you take away cylinder. Rotating the cylinder axis has no effect on spherical equivalent.
b   Plano
   "Average" spherical power of a sphero-cylindrical lens = sphere + 1/2 cylinder.

158

Question 5

For the following prescriptions determine the type and orientation of astigmatism (i.e. compound myopic, with the rule) and give the spherical equivalent.

a − 4.00 DS / + 4.00 DC axis 180
b Plano / + 2.00 DC axis 100
c − 1.00 DS / − 3.50 DC axis 10
d + 5.00 DS / − 1.00 DC axis 135
e + 2.00 DS / − 4.00 DC axis 90
f − 0.50 DS / + 4.00 DC axis 45

Answer 5

a Simple myopic astigmatism, against the rule, − 2.00 D.
b Simple hyperopic astigmatism, with the rule, + 1.00 D.
c Compound myopic astigmatism, with the rule, − 2.75 D.
d Compound hyperopic astigmatism, oblique, + 4.50 D.
e Mixed astigmatism, against the rule, plano.
f Mixed astigmatism, oblique, + 1.50 D.

Question 6

A patient reads 8 mm below the optical centres of his glasses with the following prescription:

RE − 3.00 DS   LE + 1.00 DS / + 3.00 DC axis 90

a What prismatic effect is induced in the reading position?
b Would the patient experience a right or left hyperdeviation whilst wearing these glasses in the reading position assuming no deviation in primary position?
c Is this problematic? How can it be alleviated?

Answer 6

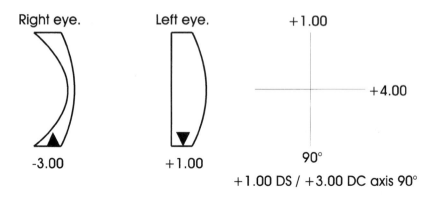

Right eye. Left eye. +1.00

-3.00 +1.00 90°

+1.00 DS / +3.00 DC axis 90°

+4.00

a 3.2Δ of vertical prism.
Calculate the prismatic power of the lenses acting in the vertical meridians using the Prentice equation:

RE 0.8 × 3.00 = 2.4Δ base down
LE 0.8 × 1.00 = 0.8Δ base up

Total prismatic effect in the reading position = 2.4 + 0.8 = 3.2Δ

RE 3.2Δ base down or LE 3.2Δ base up

b Left hyperdeviation.
Think of the effect of the lenses in deviating the visual axes as the visual axes pass from the eyes out through the lenses.

c Most patients physiologically adapt or learn to fuse small vertical deviations, but if they are symptomatic there are three options:

1 Contact lenses have a smaller prismatic effect.
2 Lowering the optical centres of both lenses will reduce the vertical imbalance between distance and near vision.
3 Slab off prism: this removes base down prism, therefore slab off the more minus or less plus lens.

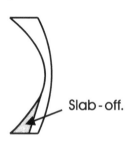

Slab - off.

Question 7

Refraction three months after corneal section extracapsular cataract surgery is shown.

plano/ − 10.00 DC axis 165

a   Transpose this prescription.
b   Is this with the rule or against the rule astigmatism? Would you remove the sutures?
c   What are the management options if after removing the sutures there is still significant astigmatism?

Answer 7

a   − 10.00 DS/ + 10.00 DC axis 75
new sphere = old sphere + old cylinder
new cylinder = same as old cylinder but change the sign
new axis = change old axis by 90 degrees
b   With the rule astigmatism; the vertical meridian has plus cylinder power. The sutures should be removed.
c   It is worth trying spectacle correction but significant astigmatism may be better corrected with a contact lens. If the patient is still symptomatic from aniseikonia or distortion they may require refractive surgery, in this instance relieving incisions on the steep axis.

Question 8

a   An eye with an amplitude of accommodation of 6 D has its near point at 50 cm.
What is the full refractive correction and where is the far point?
b   What is the range of accommodation?

Answer 8

a The refractive correction is 4.00 D of hyperopia and the far point is 25 cm behind the eye.

All 6 D of accommodation are being used at the near point of 50 cm, only 2 D focus from infinity to 50 cm, so at infinity 4 D are still active indicating 4 D of hyperopia. The far point of a 4 D hyperope is a virtual far point, i.e. 25 cm (1/4 m) behind the eye.

b Infinity to the near point at 50 cm.

The range of accommodation corresponds to the actual range of clear vision obtainable via accommodation. The 4 D used by the patient to reach infinity from the far point does not contribute to the range in this case.

Question 9

If the far point is 20 cm in front of the eye and the near point is 12.5 cm in front also, what is:

a The distance refractive correction?
b The amplitude of accommodation?
c The near point when wearing the distance correction?
d The range of accommodation when wearing the distance correction?

Answer 9

a 5.00 D of myopia.

1/far point in metres $= 1/0.2 = 5$, far point in front of the eye requires a diverging or minus lens to focus on the retina.

b 3 D.

Accommodation full at near point $1/0.125 = 8$ D
Accommodation relaxed at far point $1/0.2 = 5$ D
Amplitude of accommodation $= 8 - 5 = 3$ D

c 33 cm.

$1/3 = 0.33$ m

d Infinity to 33 cm (this is the linear extent of clear vision obtainable via accommodation).

162

Question 10

A presbyope has a range of accommodation from 5 m to 1 m. He goes without distance glasses. What power reading glasses are necessary to allow him to see clearly and comfortably at 33 cm, leaving half the accommodative amplitude in reserve?

Answer 10

2.60 D.
The amplitude of accommodation in accommodating from 5 m to 1 m.

$1/5 = 0.2$ D to $1/1 = 1$ D
i.e. 0.8 D

Half of the patient's accommodative amplitude = 0.4 D.
To see clearly 33 cm a total of $1/0.33 = 3$ D of plus power is necessary.
The patient is already 0.2 D myopic (1/far point) and he can comfortably supply 0.4 D of accommodation. Therefore the plus power of his reading glasses can be calculated:

$3.00 - 0.2 - 0.4 = 2.60$ D.

Question 11

A 20Δ prism is placed base out before the right eye of an orthophoric patient.

a Which way will the patient's right eye appear to be displaced by the examiner?
b Which way will a distant object appear to be displaced to the patient's right eye when the prism is introduced?
c What compensatory eye movement will the patient make?

Answer 11

a Nasally. The prism deviates the virtual image of the patient's eye towards its apex.

b To the patient's left. The patient sees a virtual image which is deviated towards the apex of the prism.

n.b.: the retinal image is real and is displaced temporally towards the base of the prism.

c The eye will converge. The visual axis will be directed outward by the prism, the eye will turn inwards for the image to fall on the fovea.

Clinical methods

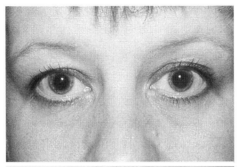

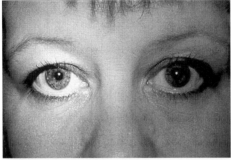

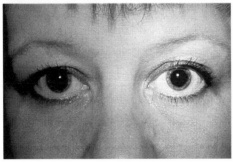

a What is this pupil abnormality?
b Where is the pathology?
c Explain the anatomical basis of this defect.
d If one pupil is mechanically or pharmacologically non-reactive is this test still relevant?
e How can a relative afferent pupillary defect be quantified?

Answer 12

a Left relative afferent pupillary defect (Marcus Gunn pupil).
b Usually an optic nerve lesion, but it can occur with gross retinal pathology. Remember that the swinging light test detects only a relative difference between the afferent pupillary reaction in the two eyes, so if both optic nerves are equally damaged a relative afferent pupillary defect will not be apparent.
c Afferent neurons from one eye reach the pretectal area, information is passed to the Edinger–Westphal nuclei bilaterally, pupillomotor information travels with the IIIrd nerve. Light stimulation of one eye, therefore, will normally result in pupil constriction of both eyes. If the afferent pathway is damaged neither pupil will constrict when light is shone into the affected side.
d Detection of an afferent pupillary defect requires only one "working" pupil; the swinging light test is performed observing the reactive pupil.
e Increasing neutral density filters are placed in front of the normal eye until the pupillary responses appear equal in the swinging light test.

Correct pupil examination

1 Room illumination must be low. If asked to test pupils in an exam, turn down the lights.
2 Instruct the patient to look in the distance. If distance fixation is not maintained, particularly if the patient looks at the light directed at the eye, the pupils will constrict as part of the near response and the light reflex cannot be assessed.
3 Be seen to use a bright flashlight. The brighter the light, the more a relative difference in the afferent pathways of the two eyes will be apparent.
4 Test the direct and consensual response of each eye in turn, then perform the swinging light test. When performing the swinging light test remember to observe each pupil for 2 or 3 seconds before swinging over to the other eye in order to detect dilatation that occurs if a relative afferent pupillary defect is present.

Question 13

a What is the diagnosis? How can you confirm this?
b What are the features?
c If you were permitted one investigation what would it be?

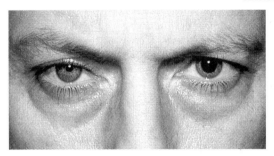

Question 13

Answer 13

a Right Horner's syndrome, oculosympathetic paralysis.

Cocaine 4% instilled into affected side will not dilate the pupil, hydroxyamphetamine 1% will dilate the pupil in a pre-ganglionic lesion but not a post-ganglionic lesion.

b Ptosis, miosis, apparent enophthalmos, anhidrosis (if anhidrosis is present this indicates the lesion is below the superior cervical ganglion), heterochromia is characteristic of congenital Horner's syndrome.

c Chest X-ray to rule out apical lung pathology, e.g. Pancoast tumour.

Question 14

a Which pupil is abnormal and why? Describe all features of this pupil abnormality.

b What is the diagnosis? What other ocular and systemic features would you look for?

c Where is the lesion?

d How could you confirm the diagnosis? Explain the mechanism.

e What investigations are indicated?

Answer 14

a The left pupil is larger than the right, the anisocoria is more apparent in bright illumination, therefore the left pupil is the abnormal one as it fails to constrict in bright light.

The left pupil has a poor direct response to light and accommodation.

b Left Adie's tonic pupil. Look for vermiform (segmental palsy) movements of the iris border at the slit lamp. Absent or diminished deep tendon reflexes with this pupil abnormality occur in the Holmes–Adie syndrome.

167

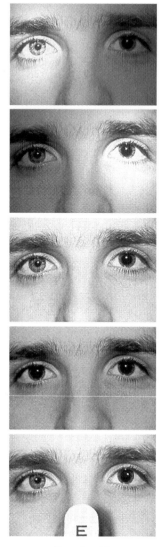

Question 14

c   Interruption of post-ganglionic ocular parasympathetic innervation to the iris sphincter muscle and ciliary muscle.
d   The abnormal pupil will constrict with pilocarpine 0.125% because of denervation hypersensitivity. This test will be falsely negative acutely as the denervation hypersensitivity takes several weeks to develop. A normal pupil will be unaffected.
e   This is a benign condition and no further investigations are indicated.

Question 15

a What is the difference between static and kinetic perimetry? Give examples of each.

b What do you understand by the island of vision?

c How far does the normal field of vision extend?

Answer 15

a Kinetic perimetry involves moving a stimulus of varying size, colour, or luminance from the periphery towards the centre to map isopters. Examples: confrontation, tangent screen, Goldmann.

In static perimetry a stimulus is presented at a predetermined position. The intensity of the target is slowly increased until it is detected by the patient, so the sensitivity of each point tested is determined. Examples: automated perimeters, Humphrey and Octopus.

b The visual field can be thought of as an "island of vision" in a sea of blindness. It is a three-dimensional structure. The peak of the island represents the point of highest visual acuity, the fovea, then it declines progressively towards the periphery. The "bottomless pit" represents the blind spot, the optic disc.

c 90 degrees temporally.
60 degrees nasally.
50 degrees superiorly.
70 degrees inferiorly.

Question 16

a What is an isopter?

b What is the difference between an absolute and relative scotoma? Give an example of a condition causing each type.

c Describe the difference between a positive and negative scotoma.

Answer 16

a An isopter encloses an area within which a target of a given size, colour, or intensity is visible. Isopters resemble the contours on a map.

b An absolute scotoma is an area within the visual field where there is total loss of vision, e.g. retinoschisis. A relative scotoma is an area where some targets can be seen but others that would normally be seen are not, e.g. retinal detachment.

c A positive scotoma is when something obstructs the central vision, e.g. macular haemorrhage, whereas a negative scotoma is when there is a "hole" in the central vision, e.g. optic nerve lesion.

Visual fields to confrontation

There are numerous methods that may be used. You must practise one method until it is second nature. Here we describe a method.

1 Each eye is tested separately. The patient covers one eye with their hand. The patient is then instructed to maintain fixation on the examiner's nose throughout the test.
2 Ask "Does my face appear clear, or are there gaps or blurred areas?". This tests the central field.
3 Test each quadrant separately by asking the patient to count fingers, then test quadrants on each side of the vertical meridian simultaneously by asking the patient to count fingers. If fingers in a given area cannot be identified correctly ask whether hand movements can be detected and map out the abnormal area by moving the hand until a normal area is reached. If an abormal area is detected, stop and repeat on the other eye.
4 If step 3 is normal ask the patient to compare the clarity of your hands which are placed on each side of the vertical meridian in first the upper and then the lower quadrants and then above and below the horizontal meridian on each side (this will detect more subtle defects). If an abnormal area is detected map it out by moving your hand until it appears clear.
5 If step 4 is normal, repeat it comparing the colour of two red targets (e.g. red top of a tropicamide bottle). If one appears desaturated compared to the other, move it to map out the abnormal area.
6 Repeat on the other eye.

Question 17

Describe the visual field defect in examples (**a**)–(**d**). Where is the lesion? Give your reasons.

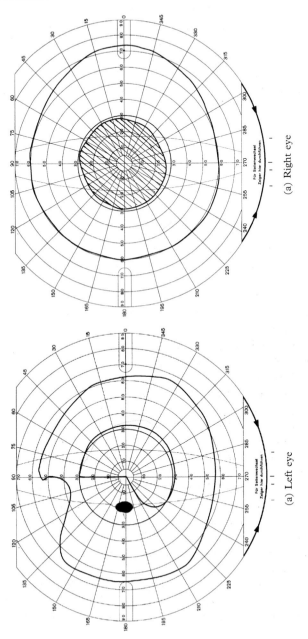

(a) Right eye

(a) Left eye

Question 17

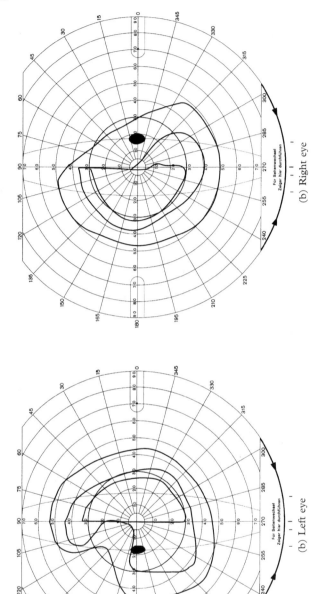

(b) Right eye

(b) Left eye

Question 17

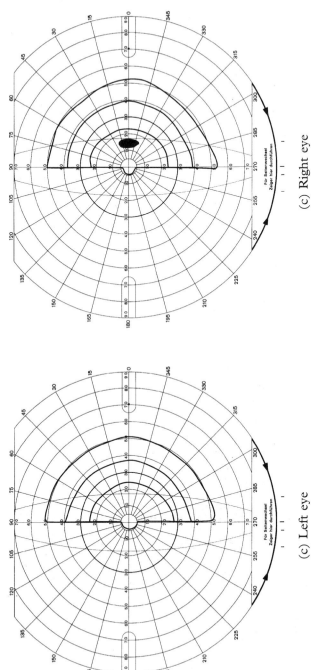

(c) Right eye

(c) Left eye

173

Question 17

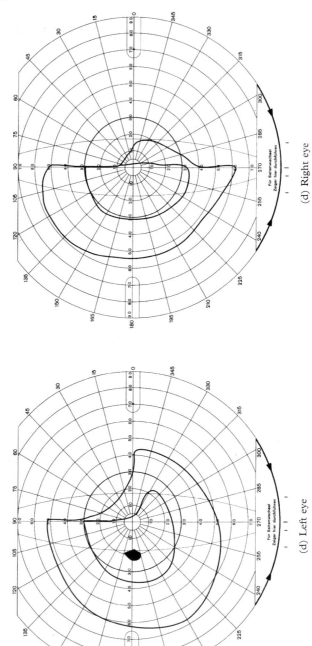

(d) Right eye

(d) Left eye

Answer 17

a Central scotoma RE, superotemporal defect LE (junctional scotoma). The lesion is at the junction of the right optic nerve and the chiasm with involvement of von Wilbrand's knee causing superotemporal loss of LE.

b Bitemporal hemianopia, affecting upper visual field.

Chiasmal lesion with compression from below, probably due to a pituitary lesion (if the inferotemporal visual field were mostly affected, the lesion would be compressing the chiasm from above, e.g. craniopharyngioma). n.b.: tilted discs can also produce this pattern of field loss.

c Left homonymous hemianopia with macular sparing.

Right occipital cortex (calcarine fissure). The macular area of the occipital visual cortex is in a watershed area with respect to blood supply (terminal branches of posterior and middle cerebral arteries). The rest of the visual field is represented by the visual cortex supplied only by the posterior cerebral artery, so loss of the posterior cerebral artery flow may mean sparing of the ipsilateral macular visual cortex because of blood supply by the middle cerebral artery.

d Right homonymous hemianopia, incongruous, denser above.

Either right optic tract or right temporal lobe; the latter is much more common than the former. This field defect is incongruous therefore the lesion is more anterior in the post-chiasmal visual pathway. (The more posterior, i.e. towards the occipital cortex, the lesion in the post-chiasmal visual pathway, the more likely the field defect is to be congruous.) The inferior retinal fibres course into the temporal lobe forming Meyer's loop. They are separated from the superior retinal fibres which course directly into the parietal lobe. Therefore superior quadrantanopias probably represent temporal lobe lesions whereas inferior quadrantanopias represent parietal lobe lesions.

Question 18

Study this visual field.

a Which indices indicate reliability of the test? Describe how the Humphrey analyser performs these tests.

b Describe this Humphrey field. What is the likely cause of the defect?

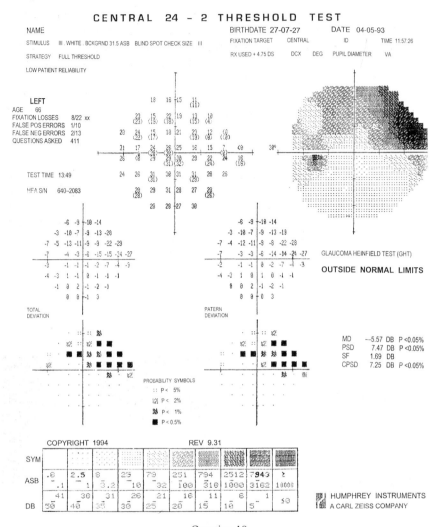

Question 18

Answer 18

a Fixation losses, false positives and false negatives, and fluctuation (SF). Fixation loss – during a test the analyser periodically checks the patient's fixation by presenting stimuli in the blind spot. If the patient responds a fixation loss is recorded.

False positive – during the test the projector moves as if to present a stimulus but does not do so. If the patient responds a false positive error is recorded.

176

False negative – at other times a stimulus which is much brighter than threshold is presented in an area where sensitivity has already been determined. If the patient does not respond, a false negative is recorded. Fluctuation – threshold is determined twice at ten predetermined point locations. Fluctuation is calculated on the basis of the differences between the first and second measurements at each of the ten points.

b There is low patient reliability with greater than 20% fixation losses (XX indicates this). The gray scale shows a superior field defect of the left eye which is most dense nasally and appears to extend to the blind spot (superior arcuate scotoma). The total deviation plot represents the difference between the patient and age-corrected normal, here it shows a high probability (<0.5%) that this is a true defect. The pattern deviation plot has the same high probability in these areas. The pattern deviation plot adjusts for any shift in overall sensitivity (e.g. cataract or small pupil), therefore in this patient there is focal loss in this area. The likely cause of this field defect is glaucoma.

Question 19

(a)   (b)

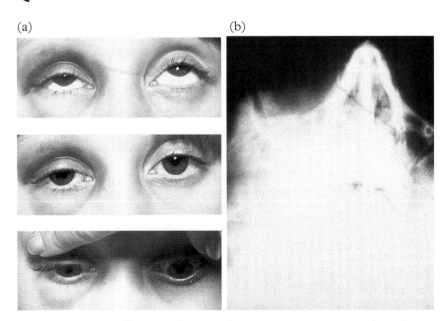

a Describe the eye movements shown here.
b Describe the X-ray findings shown. What is the diagnosis?
c What problems may this patient encounter?
d Which tests are useful in monitoring this condition?

Answer 19

a Minimal right hypotropia in primary position (look at corneal reflexes). Moderate limitation of right depression and marked limitation of right elevation.

b Opaque right maxillary sinus. Step and linear break in the inferior orbital rim, this is typical of an orbital floor or blow-out fracture. (Other X-ray features seen are fluid level in the maxillary sinus on the affected side and entrapment of orbital tissues in the floor of the orbit visible in the maxillary sinus; the "tear drop" sign.)

c Diplopia, usually vertical separation (horizontal separation if there is an ethmoidal fracture in the medial wall of the orbit also). Diplopia reverses from looking up to looking down. Reading may be difficult.

d Hess chart and field of BSV (binocular single vision) (*see* Question 33 *below*).

Question 20

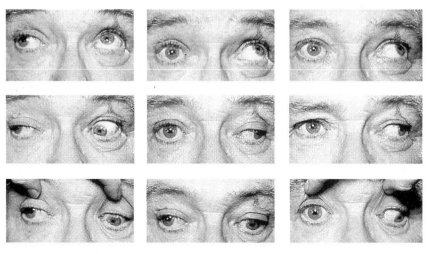

a Describe this patient's ocular movements.

b What is the diagnosis? What else would you want to examine?

c What is the significance of pupil involvement?

d How do you test the IVth cranial nerve in this situation?

e Describe the abnormality in this CT scan. What specific symptom will you ask about if you are thinking about this diagnosis as a cause for this patient's signs?

f What investigations other than CT scan will you perform and why?

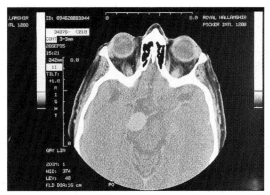

Question 20e

Answer 20

a In primary position the left eye is deviated outwards, the patient is fixing with the right eye, there is marked restriction of the right eye in elevation and adduction and a lesser degree of reduced depression. It is difficult to be sure whether there is a degree of right ptosis as there has been obvious trauma over the left upper eyelid causing left ptosis and a scar, but there is an impression of elevation of the right upper eyelid on adduction (inverse Duane's syndrome).

b Right IIIrd nerve palsy, with possible aberrant regeneration. Examine for pupil involvement. Also examine other cranial nerves as well as a full neurological examination to ascertain the site of the lesion.

c The pupillary fibres travel superficially in the IIIrd nerve, which leaves them more susceptible to external compression than to the effects of an intrinsic nerve lesion from vascular infarction. So a IIIrd nerve palsy caused by a compressive lesion, such as an aneurysm or a tumour, is likely to have pupil involvement, whereas an ischaemic IIIrd nerve palsy from microvascular disease is likely to spare the pupil.

d Look for intorsion of the globe on attempted downgaze. If this occurs the IVth nerve is intact.

e This CT is enhanced with contrast ("cont" documented top left hand corner). An area of oval shaped increased attenuation can be seen in the area of the circle of Willis on the right. This is a posterior communicating artery aneurysm. It is important to ask about pain as sudden enlargement of the aneurysmal sac by haemorrhage often causes a painful IIIrd nerve paresis with pupillary involvement.

f Blood pressure and blood glucose: hypertension and diabetes are common causes of a microvascular IIIrd nerve palsy (pupil sparing).
ESR: vasculitis due to giant cell arteritis, SLE, and PAN (systemic lupus erythematosus, polyarteritis nodosa).
FBC: may indicate systemic pathology.
Autoantibodies: looking for a vasculitic process.

179

Question 21

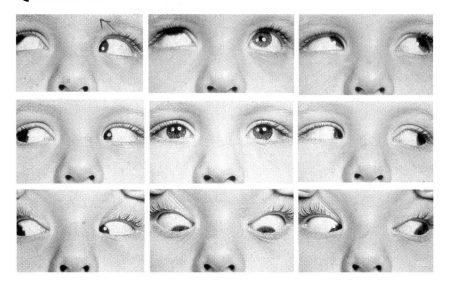

a Describe this patient's ocular movements.
b What is the diagnosis? How might you confirm this?
c What is the differential diagnosis?

Answer 21

a The eyes are straight in primary position. There is limited elevation of the left eye, especially in adduction with near normal elevation in abduction. There is overaction of the contralateral (right) superior rectus, but no other muscle sequelae.
b Left Brown's or superior oblique tendon sheath syndrome. A forced duction test will be positive when attempting to elevate the eye from the adducted position.
c Isolated inferior oblique under-action, but this is rare.

Question 22

a Describe this patient's eye movements,
b Describe the abnormal head posture this patient may have.
c Describe the possible aetiology of this pattern of eye movements.
d List the specific conditions this pattern may be associated with.

180

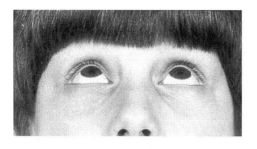

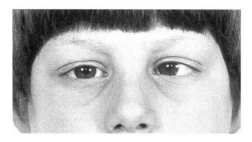

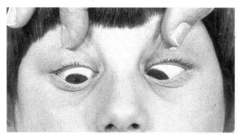

Question 22

Answer 22

a In primary position there is a left esotropia, on downgaze this esodeviation is significantly increased whereas on upgaze the eyes appear straight. This is a "V" eso pattern. Diagnosis is based on a minimum difference of 15Δ from upgaze to downgaze.

b Chin down.

c Lateral rectus overaction resulting in more abduction on elevation.
High medial rectus insertions resulting in more adduction on depression.
Superior oblique underaction resulting in less abduction on depression.
Inferior oblique overaction resulting in more abduction on elevation.

d Infantile esotropia, Duane's syndrome, Brown's syndrome, acquired bilateral IVth cranial nerve palsy.

181

Question 23

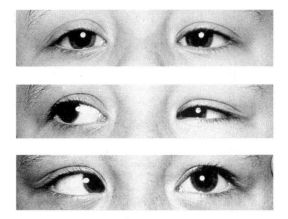

a Describe this patient's eye movements. What is the diagnosis?
b Which eye is more commonly affected by this syndrome?
c List ocular and systemic abnormalities associated with this syndrome.
d What compensatory head posture may this patient adopt?
e Give a classification of abnormal head posture.

Answer 23

a In primary position there is a small angle left esotropia, on left gaze there is marked reduction of the left eye in abduction, the left eye does not abduct beyond the midline, and on looking to the right the palpebral aperture of the left eye narrows but it appears to adduct fully. The right eye abducts and adducts fully with no change in the palpebral aperture.

   This is left Duane's syndrome.
b Left.
c Ocular: colobomata, iris heterochromia, lens opacities, microphthalmia, persistent pupillary membrane.

   General: Goldenhar's and Klippel–Feil syndromes.
d This patient may adopt a face turn to the affected side, the left. This head posture is adopted to centralize a small field of binocular fixation.
e Classification may be related to causes of abnormal head posture.
   Non-ocular head posture: torticollis, deafness, defect of balance, habit.
   Ocular head postures: obtain/maintain BSV and place it centrally, e.g. mechanical restriction of movement; obtain better vision, e.g. nystagmus, ptosis.

Question 24

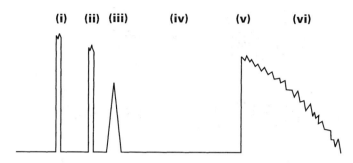

(i)   (ii) (iii)   (iv)   (v)   (vi)

a What does "A" stand for in A-scan?

b The diagram shows an axial A-scan of a normal eye (contact method). What structure does each number represent?

c What is the most common indication for A-scan? Are there any other indications for axial eye-length measurement?

d What effect does silicone oil have on A-scan axial length measurement and why?

Answer 24

a Amplitude

b (i)   cornea
   (ii)   anterior lens surface/iris
   (iii) posterior lens surface
   (iv) vitreous
   (v)   retina
   (vi) orbital contents

c Measuring axial length for biometry calculation. Other indications include looking for posterior staphyloma, diagnosing axial myopia as a cause of pseudo-proptosis, diagnosing nanophthalmos and microphthalmia.

d It gives a falsely long axial length because sound velocity is significantly reduced in silicone oil compared to aqueous or vitreous.

Question 25

a   What does "B" stand for in B-scan?

b   How do B-scans differ from A-scans?

c   At what frequency do standardised B-scans emit the focused sound beam?

d   Describe the ocular abnormality shown. What other investigations confirm the diagnosis? Why is this diagnosis important to make?

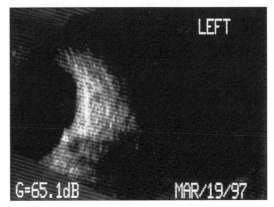

e   Describe the ocular abnormalities shown in (e).

Answer 25

a   Brightness.

b   A-scans produce a one-dimensional image making measurement of thickness of structures and length between them possible. B-scans produce a two-dimensional slice of tissue images, making it possible to look at anatomical relationships in and around the eye.

c   10 Hz.

d   In this low gain scan there is an obvious signal at the optic nerve head; this is typical of disc drusen. Optic nerve head drusen show the phenomenon of autofluorescence and they can be imaged on CT scan. It is important to make this diagnosis in patients with pseudo-papilloedema avoiding unnecessary investigation.

e   (i)   Retinal detachment; membranous opacity inserted into the optic nerve head. (n.b.: PVD has no attachment to the optic nerve.)

(ii)   Posterior scleritis; area of low reflectivity between outer sclerea and orbital fat (Tenon's space) and thickening of the globe wall. The inflammation spreads to the optic nerve sheath giving the "T-sign".

(iii)   Choroidal melanoma; mushroom/collar stud mass. (Other features may include choroidal excavation and associated retinal detachment.)

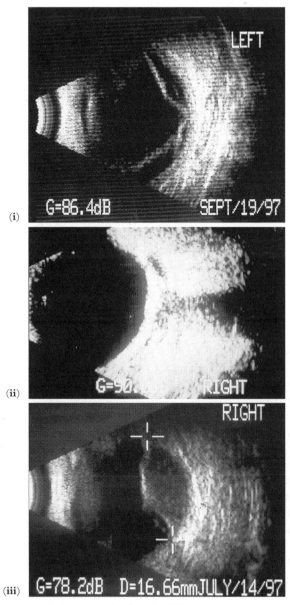

(i)

(ii)

(iii)

Question 25e

185

Question 26

Regarding physical properties of fluorescein and features of fundus fluorescein angiography:

a What is the molecular weight?
b What percentage is protein bound?
c How is it excreted?
d What is the efficiency of fluorescence?
e Give the wavelengths of excitation and emission.
f What are the phases of a normal fluorescein angiogram?
g What are the mechanisms of hypofluorescence? Give examples.
h What are the mechanisms of hyperfluorescence? Give examples.

Answer 26

a 376.
b 80% (significant free fluorescein).
c Renal.
d 100%.
e 485 nm and 530 nm.
f Choroidal phase (pre-arterial), arterial phase (6–8 seconds), arteriovenous phase, venous phase, and late phase.
g Masking by excess pigment, e.g. melanin in choroidal naevus, blood in choroidal haemorrhage; masking by fluid in subretinal space, e.g. central serous retinopathy; filling defects, occlusion of blood vessels of choroid or retina.
h Transmission/window defects, e.g. lack of pigment RPE atrophy; abnormal blood vessels which leak, e.g. new vessels, choroidal neovascular membrane; pooling and staining, e.g. pooling in CSR, staining of drusen.

Question 27

Describe the abnormal finding in these FFAs and give the diagnosis.

Question 27

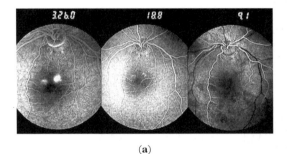

(a)

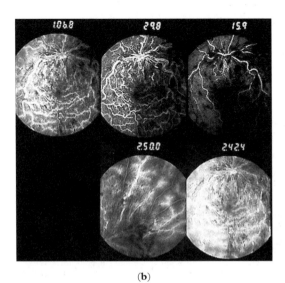

(b)

Answer 27

a The arterial phase shows patchy choroidal filling and a hint of masking
in the inferior macular area corresponding to a serous detachment. The
later phases show two areas of hyperfluorescence due to leakage which
increase in size and there is more obvious masking by the serous
detachment. This is a typical central serous retinopathy (CSR).

b Early phase shows normal arterial circulation and masking of background fluorescence by haemorrhages. Capillaries and veins are slow
to fill. The later phase shows marked dilatation and tortuosity of the
retinal veins with staining of the venous walls and leakage from the
optic disc. The last film in the series shows marked capillary non-
perfusion. This is an ischaemic central retinal vein occlusion.

187

Question 28

Regarding the physical properties of indocyanine green and indocyanine green angiography:

a   What is the molecular weight?
b   What percentage is protein bound?
c   How is it excreted?
d   What is the efficiency of fluorescence?
e   Give the wavelengths of excitation and emission.
f   Explain the main differences between fluorescein angiography and indocyanine green angiography with particular reference to the different properties of the two dyes.

Answer 28

a   775.
b   98% (insignificant free indocyanine).
c   Hepatic.
d   4% (inefficient fluorescence).
e   805 nm and 835 nm.
f   (i)   Indocyanine green (ICG) is highly protein bound compared to fluorescein, therefore it does (not) escape from the fenestrated choriocapillaris and obscure underlying choroidal detail, unlike fluorescein.
   (ii)   The efficient first pass effect in the liver of ICG limits the recirculation phenomenon which occurs with fluorescein angiography.
   (iii)   The spectral absorption and emission characteristics of ICG permit visualisation of the choroid which is not visible in fluorescein angiography.
   (iv)   ICG transit is very rapid compared to fluorescein so ICG angiography does not have the characteristic phases of fluorescein angiography.

Question 29

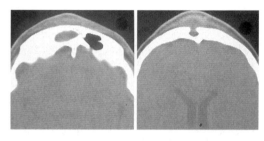

(a)

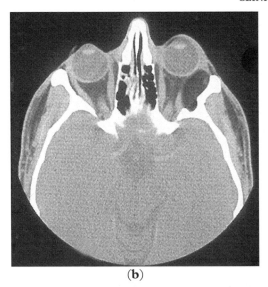

(b)

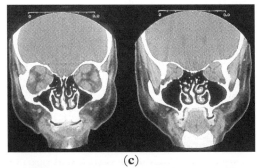

(c)

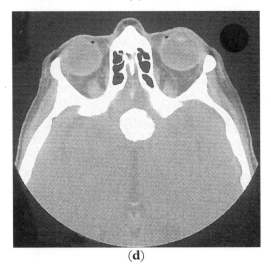

(d)

Describe the abnormalities in the CT scans shown and give the likely diagnosis.

Answer 29

a There is a soft tissue swelling over the forehead. The right frontal sinus is filled with soft tissue material and in one point the outer cortex is breached. There is no evidence of intracranial involvement in these sections. The most likely diagnosis is a mucocoele of the right frontal sinus which has eroded the outer vault.

b There is a large, well-defined, low density area lying within the left orbit. It is extraconal but is displacing the lateral rectus medially and is causing erosion of the lateral wall of the orbit, especially posteriorly. The bone erosion suggests the lesion is longstanding. There is left proptosis. The density of the lesion is of a fatty nature and the most likely diagnosis is an intra-orbital dermoid.

c This coronal section shows severe bilateral enlargement of the ocular extra-ocular muscles. There is gross compression of the optic nerves in the orbital apices. This is severe dysthroid ophthalmopathy.

d This axial section shows a densely calcified mass in the chiasmal area (only single axial section shown, therefore difficult to localise accurately). This is the appearance of a densely calcified meningioma.

Question 30

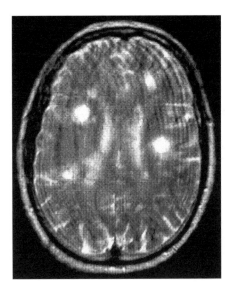

a Describe the abnormality on this MRI, what is the likely diagnosis?
b Is CT or MRI more sensitive in this disease?

Answer 30

a There are multiple large foci of high signal within the white matter of both hemispheres. These appearances are consistent with demyelination.
b MRI. Constrast enhanced CT will show white matter lesions in 25% of patients with clinically diagnosed multiple sclerosis and recent symptoms, whereas MRI will show white matter disease in 90% of these patients. T_2 weighted images are particularly sensitive at detecting these lesions relative to surrounding brain.

Question 31

Look at the Hess chart.

a Which eye has the under-acting muscle? Explain your reasoning.
b What is the probable diagnosis?
c On what principles is the Hess chart based?

Answer 31

a Right. The eye with the smaller field is the eye with the primary limitation of movement.
b Right lateral rectus palsy (VIth nerve). Maximum inward displacement of the dots occurs in the direction of the main action of the affected muscle.
c The principles of the Hess chart are Hering's and Sherrington's laws of innervation, dissociation of the eyes with complementary colours (Hess) or a mirror (Lees screen) and foveal projection.

Question 32

Look at the Hess charts.

a Which is the under-acting muscle in (**a**)?
b Chart (**b**) shows the same patient after several months. What does it demonstrate?

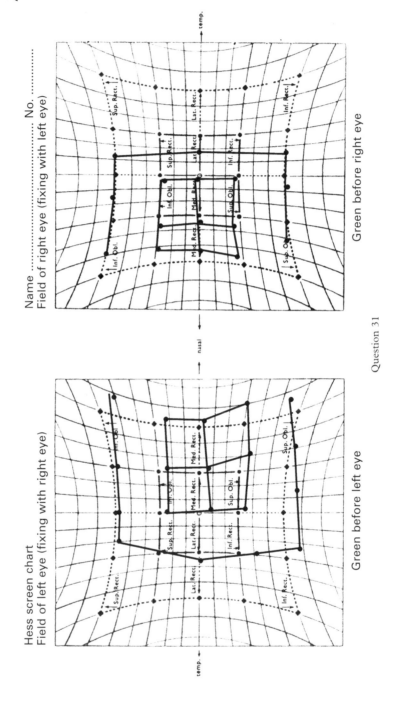

Question 31

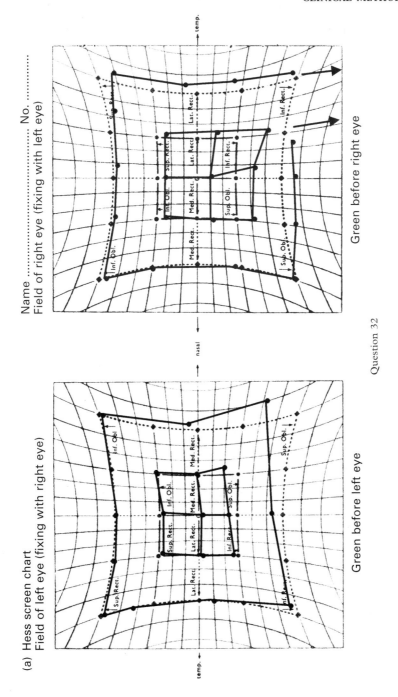

(a) Hess screen chart

Field of right eye (fixing with left eye)

Name .... No. ....

Green before right eye

Field of left eye (fixing with right eye)

Green before left eye

Question 32

193

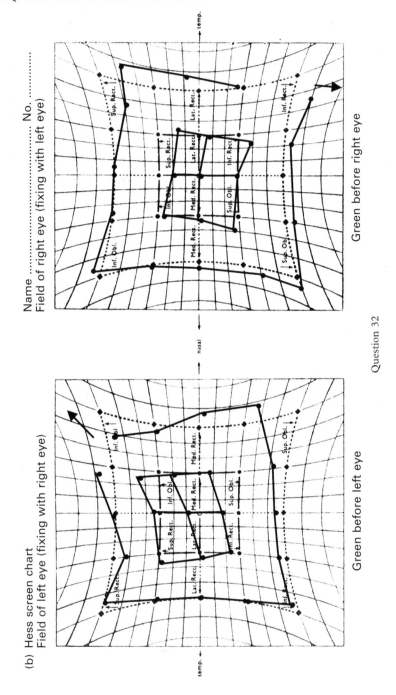

(b) Hess screen chart

Question 32

Answer 32

a The left superior oblique. The left eye has the smaller central field and the largest inward displacement of dots occurs in the field of action of the superior oblique.

b This chart demonstrates the muscle sequelae of a left IVth nerve palsy: right inferior rectus over-action (over-action of the contralateral synergist); left inferior oblique over-action (contracture of the ipsilateral antagonist); right superior rectus under-action (secondary inhibitional palsy of contralateral antagonist). Outward displacement of the dots occurs in the field of action of an over-acting muscle.

Question 33

a Describe the abnormality in the Hess chart.
b Is it typical of mechanical or neurogenic restriction? What feature points you to your choice?
c What is the likely diagnosis?

Answer 33

a The right eye has marked limitation of elevation and depression, producing a compressed field.
b This is mechanical restriction; typically the affected eye has a narrow field in opposing directions of movement.
c Right orbital floor fracture.

Question 34

Study this orthoptic report.

Patient wearing　　　$+4.50\,DS/ - 0.50\,DC \times 90$　　　$+3.50\,DS$
(full refractive correction minus the working distance)

Visual acuity
with glasses	6/12	6/6
	N6	N5

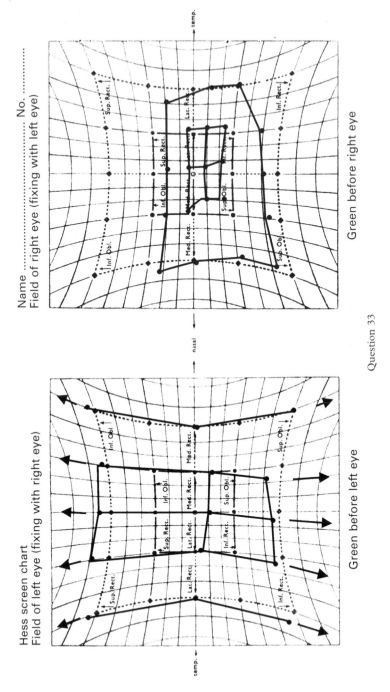

Name .... No. ....
Field of right eye (fixing with left eye)

Green before right eye

Hess screen chart
Field of left eye (fixing with right eye)

Green before left eye

Question 33

Cover test

with glasses	1/3 m slight esophoria with good recovery
	6 m minimal esophoria with good recovery
without glasses	1/3 m ⎫ occasionally straight to light ⇒ moderate
	6 m ⎭ right esotropia on accommodation

Ocular movements full

Convergence

with glasses   binocular to nose

Bagolini glasses

with glasses	1/3 m ⎫ BSV response without manifest deviation
	6 m ⎭
without glasses	1/3 m ⎫ right suppression with right esotropia
	6 m ⎭

Prism fusion range

with glasses	1/3 m BO 35Δ BI 8Δ
	6 m BO 18Δ BI 2Δ
without glasses	nil fusion as manifest

Wirt

| with glasses | positive to fly |
| | circles 140 seconds of arc |

4 dioptre prism test positive for right central suppression

Prism cover test

with glasses	1/3 m esophoria 6Δ
	6 m esophoria 2Δ
without glasses	1/3 m right esotropia 35Δ
	6 m right esotropia 30Δ

AC/A ratio   7:1

Binocular visual acuity

with glasses	1/3 m	6/12
	6 m	6/12
without glasses	1/3 m	nil
	6 m	nil

a Describe this patient's strabismus.
b Explain why the right visual acuity is reduced.
c Describe the grades of binocular vision.
d What is the Bagolini glasses test?
e What is the principle of the Wirt test? Describe another principle used in testing stereopsis and give an example.
f What is the normal horizontal prism fusion range?

g What is the 4 dioptre prism test?

h What is the AC/A ratio? Describe the two methods of measuring it. What is the normal AC/A ratio?

i What is meant by binocular visual acuity (BVA)? Does the level of BVA achieved by this patient surprise you?

Answer 34

a Right fully accommodative esotropia. Without glasses the cover test reveals a right esotropia, the near and distance angles are almost the same. With full hypermetropic correction the cover test reveals a small degree of esophoria with good recovery.

b The right eye is amblyopic due to anisometropia.

c Worth's classification of binocular vision: (1) simultaneous perception, (2) fusion, (3) stereopsis.

d This test investigates retinal correspondence. Bagolini eye pieces each incorporate fine parallel striations, one side at 45 degrees the other at 135 degrees. A spotlight viewed through the glass produces a line image. The patient is asked how many line images and spotlights are seen and what form the lines make. The pattern seen corresponds to the type of retinal correspondence (bifoveal or abnormal), and degrees of suppression. In this patient a symmetrical cross centred on the spotlight indicates binocular single vision. Normal or abnormal retinal correspondence will give this result; the latter can be differentiated from the former by cover test – abnormal retinal correspondence will have a manifest deviation on cover test.

e The Wirt or Titmus stereotest is based on linear polarization and consists of two plates. One plate contains the image of a fly: if the wings stand out from the body gross stereopsis is present. The second plate consists of nine boxes each containing circles, and three rows of animals. Stereopsis up to 40 seconds of arc may be achieved.

The TNO stereotest uses the principle of random dot stereograms.

f The normal horizontal prism fusion range:
Near: 35/40 prism dioptres base out and 16 prism dioptres base in.
Distance: 16 prism dioptres base out and 8 prism dioptres base in.

g This test assesses the presence of bifoveal fixation. If normal bifoveal fixation is present, on placing a 4 dioptre prism base out in front of the right eye, both eyes will make a conjugate movement to the left, then a subsequent disconjugate fusional movement of the left eye will be seen. A prism placed in front of the left eye will produce a similar fusional movement, but in the opposite direction. The patient in this report has a right central suppression scotoma demonstrated by this test. When the prism is placed in front of the left eye a conjugate movement will be seen to the right, but no disconjugate fusional movement will be seen in the affected right eye because the image has been displaced into the suppression scotoma. When the prism is placed in front of the affected right eye no movement is seen in either eye because the image is already within the suppression scotoma.

h Accommodative convergence/accommodation ratio: it represents the amount of accommodative convergence exerted in response to one unit of accommodation. The normal ratio is 4/1 or slightly lower.

The AC/A ratio is measured by changing the stimulus to accommodation and assessing the amount of accommodative convergence which results from this change. The heterophoria method changes the distance of the fixation target from infinity to 33 cm, and the gradient method uses spherical lenses to increase or decrease the amount of accommodation.

i Binocular visual acuity describes the maximum visual acuity achieved while maintaining binocular single vision.

This patient achieves 6/12 BVA; this is to be expected, as 6/12 is the best visual acuity of the right eye. BVA will not be better than the weaker eye.

Part Three

Practical Methods

Steps in refraction

This is a typical routine that can be modified to suit the individual patient. More advanced techniques (such as binocular refraction, dynamic crossed cylinder) have not been included. When learning to refract, it is often helpful to sit in on an experienced refractionist (a local optometrist may be willing for you to spend some time in their practice), and to practise the techniques on a wide range of patients.

History and symptoms

- Ascertain whether the patient has an amblyopic ("lazy") eye, or a squint, and ask about family history.
- Ask how old the current spectacles are, and about the particular problems the patient is having.
- Look through the records for any previous refractive details, and try to ascertain how the refraction has been altering over the years.
- By relating the patient's history to their refractive status, a change in refraction becomes obvious, e.g. the onset of presbyopia, an increase in myopia.

Preliminary examination

- Measure visual acuities (with the appropriate correction in place). Keep this figure in mind during the examination; if the visual acuity with your refractive result is significantly better than with the current spectacles, a change of glasses may be indicated. If VA is below 6/6 with the current spectacles, the pinhole can be used – an improvement with the pinhole suggests refractive error, or media opacities. Unaided acuities can help indicate the extent of a refractive error.
- Perform a cover test, and tests of ocular motor balance and convergence. Note whether the patient has a squint.

Retinoscopy

- Dim the room lights.
- Place working distance lenses in front of both eyes, and perform retinoscopy. If the patient is obviously a myope, it is quicker to start with no lenses in the trial frame. If you have a record of the previous prescription, or access to the patient's glasses, it is quicker to start with a spherical lens equal to the spherical component of the prescription plus your working distance lens in place. For a hypermetrope, check that sufficient plus lens power is in place in front of both eyes by sweeping the retinoscope across both eyes – if you see a slow with movement, insert more plus power to ensure that the patient is not being stimulated to accommodate.
- Remember that unless the patient is presbyopic or cycloplegia is used, it is important to relax the patient's accommodation by directing their gaze to a distance fixation point (the duochrome or a spotlight works well). Sit near the visual axis of the eye under examination whilst ensuring that the patient can still see the distance fixation point.
- If the patient has a squint occlude the opposite eye so that retinoscopy is always performed close to the visual axis (to avoid oblique astigmatism). In a non-strabismic patient leaving both eyes unoccluded will help ensure that the patient does not converge (and accommodate).

Check sphere power

Following retinoscopy, put the room lights on, occlude the opposite eye, and check acuity. Two common methods of checking the sphere power at this stage are:

- Duochrome. This only works well if the patient has good VA (6/9 or better). The end point is when the letters (or circles) on the red background are clearer than those on the green, and an extra $-0.50\,\text{DS}$ makes the letters on the green background clearest. For young patients, and hypermetropes, it is acceptable to leave the patient balanced (red and green equally clear), or with the green clearest – accommodation will be stimulated under these circumstances. If there is not $0.50\,\text{DS}$ interval between red and green on the duochrome test, it is best to abandon the duochrome. The duochrome is less reliable and more difficult to use in the presence of active accommodation (e.g. children), uncorrected astigmatism, a large or small pupil, media opacities, and colour vision anomalies.
- Optimising sphere power by changing lenses, and asking the patient to report which is clearest. The aim is to leave the patient with the most

positive lens power that gives the best visual acuity. Work in 0.25 or 0.50 steps, depending on the patient's acuity. The patient has to look at the smallest letters that they can read, and a small change of sphere power is inserted in the trial frame. Always start with additional plus power before trying minus power, otherwise the patient may accommodate and confuse the result. Remember that a plus lens will either have little noticeable effect on acuity (if the patient was previously being forced to accommodate) or it will make things blurred (if there was already sufficient, or too much plus power in place). A minus lens will typically either have little noticeable effect (if the previous lens was correct, or if too much minus lens power was already in place), or it will make things clearer (if there was too much plus power in place). If the patient reports that the letters look smaller when a low powered minus lens is added to the trial frame, they are being forced to accommodate with the new lens.

Check cylinder axis and power
(crossed-cylinder technique)

- Insert an extra −0.25 or −0.50 DS to stimulate accommodation. When accommodation is active, it may be assumed that the circle of least confusion will be focused on the retina.
- Direct the patient to look at a circular letter near their acuity limit. Always check axis before power.
- To check the axis, place the handle of the crossed cylinder along the axis of the trial case cylinder, and twirl the lens. If the patient prefers one position over the other move the trial case cylinder towards the plus axis (if using plus cylinders) of the crossed cylinder when it is in the preferred position. The end point is achieved when both positions are equally blurred.
- To check power, position the crossed cylinder with one axis on top of the axis of the trial frame cylinder, and twirl the lens. If the patient prefers one position over the other, adjust the power of the cylinder so that (using plus cylinders) if the plus axis of the crossed cylinder is on top of the trial frame cylinder, power should be increased. Change power in 0.25 DC or 0.50 DC steps. The end point is reached when both positions of the crossed cylinder are equally blurred. If the cylinder power is changed by 0.50 DC, change the sphere power by 0.25 DS in the opposite direction to keep the patient's accommodation stable (therefore, if cylinder power is changed by +0.50 DC, change sphere power by −0.25 DS). If the power is altered, re-check the axis.

205

Re-check sphere power

Use lenses or duochrome.

Repeat the tests on the other eye

Binocular tests

- Once both eyes have been refracted, remove the occluder from the trial frame and direct the patient's vision towards the smallest letters they can read. (If they report diplopia, wait for a minute or so to see if they can fuse the images. If not, further investigation is required. It may be that prolonged occlusion has dissociated a large phoria, or the prescription may be causing the problem.)
- Binocular balancing – the Humphriss method is described here. Blur the left eye using a $+0.75$ DS or $+1.00$ DS lens (use the higher power if you are not confident in your refraction). This will allow you to check the sphere power of the right eye while vergence is reasonably well controlled. Once the right eye has been checked, swap the fogging lens to the right eye, and check the left eye. Binocular balancing is not possible if the patient has a squint, significantly different acuities, or a large phoria.
- Binocular addition. Once the prescription is balanced, place $+0.25$ DS in front of both eyes, and ask the patient whether the smallest letters they can see are still clear. If the prescription is correct, the letters will blur with the additional plus power. If not, incorporate the extra positive power and repeat the test. Very rarely, minus lens power will improve acuity.

Ocular motor balance

Measure and record the patient's phoria using the cover test or Maddox rod. If there is a likelihood of the phoria breaking down, consider modifying the prescription, or incorporating prisms.

Near tests

- The need for a reading prescription should be established. Is the patient of presbyopic age? Do they suffer symptoms of presbyopia?
- Check accommodation monocularly and binocularly (use the RAF rule). Amplitudes should be nearly equal in each eye. If a reading addition is

required, use the patient's age as a guide to the initial lens, or calculate from the formula:

addition = working distance (in dioptres) − 0.5 (amplitude)

Therefore, if the working distance is 3 D (33 cm), and the patient has an amplitude of 4 D, the initial addition would be +1 DS. This is placed in the trial frame, and near acuity checked. Adjust the lens power by:

- Near duochrome (if available) – detail should be clearest on the green, and +0.50 DS should make detail clearest on the red.
- Checking the range of clear vision – using small print, check that the patient can read comfortably at their desired working distance. The ideal lens will give a slightly bigger range of clear vision behind the working position.

Check ocular motor balance

Do this in the near position using the cover test or Maddox wing whilst the reading prescription is in place.

Prescribing

Prescribe new spectacles if the patient has symptoms that would be expected to be relieved by using glasses, or if there is noticeable (to the patient) improvement in vision with the new prescription compared to their current situation. Relate the patient's needs to the prescription – for example, a small distance prescription may be worthwhile for driving (a tiny prescription may be worthwhile for critical occupations such as pilots).

Notes

- Do not forget that the pinhole test is a very useful way of checking for the presence of refractive error, and can be used at any stage of the refraction.
- Patients with small pupils will have an increased depth of focus, and can be expected to be less aware of blur than those with large pupils.
- The +1 test is a quick check of sphere power. If the patient's acuity is 6/5–6/6, +1 DS blur should reduce acuity to approximately 6/12–6/18.
- A common mistake is to give too high a reading addition, forcing the patient to hold things close.
- For any large change of prescription, particularly astigmatism or anisometropia, the patient should be warned of possible symptoms in the new spectacles.

Keratometry

Uses

Keratometers are designed to measure the curvature of the anterior corneal surface. They are commonly used in biometry of the eye, and for contact lens fitting. Other uses include recognition of distortion of the corneal surface (e.g. in keratoconus), and checking the radii of curvature of contact lenses.

Optical principle of the keratometer

The cornea is considered to act as a convex mirror.

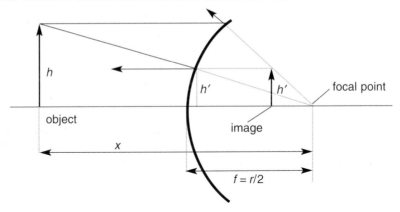

For a spherical convex mirror with radius of curvature r, if an object of height h is placed a distance x from the focal point of the mirror, the height of the image (h') can be calculated from the equation:

$$h'/h = (r/2) / x$$

This equation can be rearranged to find r:

$$r = (2x \cdot h') / h$$

For keratometers, only very small errors are introduced if x is considered to be constant. This is because the distance between the object and the image is fixed, and as the object distance is large, the image is formed very near the focal point. Therefore, keratometers are used at a fixed distance from the cornea. This makes focusing the eye piece of importance (see later), as otherwise an incorrect distance will be used. Then, if an object of fixed size is used (as in the Helmholtz keratometer) the equation becomes:

$$r = h' \text{ . constant}$$

and corneal curvature is found by measuring the size of the image.

Alternatively, for a fixed size of image (as in the Javal–Schiotz keratometer), the curvature is found by altering the size of the object since:

$$r = \text{constant} / h$$

The small image (a few millimetres) is viewed with a compound microscope, and since both designs rely on a measurement of the size of this image, any eye would also be magnified, making the technique difficult. This is overcome by optical "doubling" of the image, so that the image is optically shifted until it is just in contact with its double. The height of the image is then equal to the amount of doubling, and since both images move together when the eye moves, both stay in register. The Helmholtz design uses variable doubling so that different image sizes can be measured. The Javal–Schiotz uses a fixed amount of doubling, and the object size is varied to achieve the correct position of the images.

The scale of a keratometer gives the radius in millimetres, or the refractive power of the entire cornea in dioptres. For the conversion to dioptres, the refractive index is often assumed to be 1.3375 (1.332 to 1.338 depending on the manufacturer). The value takes into account the negative power of the posterior surface of the cornea.

One-and two-position designs

The axes of a toric surface are perpendicular, and once one meridian has been measured the instrument is rotated around to measure the other meridian (two-position design). Some variable doubling keratometers use a large, circular mire (object), and the doubling can be varied in two perpendicular directions (e.g. Bausch and Lomb). Then, the instrument is aligned with one meridian of the cornea, and both meridians can be measured without rotating the instrument. Although quicker to use, such one-position instruments do not allow accurate measurements of corneas with irregular astigmatism.

How to use keratometers

- Dim the lights to improve the visibility of the rather dim reflections from the cornea.
- Most keratometers have an eye piece graticule to aid focusing – unscrew the eye piece and then slowly screw it in until the visible scale is just focused. This relaxes the observer's accommodation. Failure to do so may give rise to significant errors on many keratometers.
- Seat the patient at the correct height, with their chin on the rest and forehead steadied against the forehead rest. If fitted with an occluder, covering the opposite eye of the patient will discourage excess convergence.
- Instruct the patient to look into the centre of the instrument (many have a small fixation light in the middle). Incorrect fixation can give rise to significant errors.
- Adjust the distance of the instrument until the images of the mires are clearly focused.
- Find the principal axis to be measured by rotating the instrument until the mires are in alignment.
- Alter the doubling (or the separation of the objects) until the correct configuration of the image is seen.
- Read off the scale – most corneal radii are in the range 6.00–9.00 mm.
- If astigmatism is present, note the astigmatic axis:
  two-position instruments – rotate the instrument to the other axis (approximately 90 degrees in most cases) and take another reading;
  one-position instruments – vary the doubling until the mires are aligned in both directions.
- If accuracy is vital (e.g. during biometry), take the mean of three or more readings.

It is possible to increase the range of the Javal–Schiotz type of keratometer using lenses between the microscope and the patient's eye, to measure concave surfaces (such as contact lenses), and to assess corneal shape across the cornea (largely redundant if a corneal topographer is available). These uses of the keratometer are outside the scope of this book.

Accuracy and errors

The design of the keratometer relies on approximations which are largely overcome by calibrating the instrument on steel ball bearings of known radius. Most instruments can be expected to be accurate to within 0.50 D, and to give reproducible results. Keratometers measure curvature at a point in an annulus of radius approximately 1.5 mm (depending on the keratometer design) centred on the visual axis. As the cornea is not a spherical surface, its radius may be different at the corneal apex. Again, this may be partly taken account of in the calibration, but inaccuracies will arise if the patient does not fixate centrally. If the eyepiece is not calibrated, errors of the order of $+/-0.1$ mm can occur. Finally, since different keratometers may use different refractive indices to calculate corneal power, it makes sense to quote radius rather than power, so that a comparison is possible with measurements taken on a different instrument.

Measurement of inter-pupillary distance (IPD)

During refraction, patients should view through the optical centres of the trial lenses, so that prismatic effects and aberrations are minimised. When spectacles are prescribed, the same considerations apply. In practice, the importance of IPD measurement depends slightly on the strength of the refractive correction, and must be as accurate as possible for higher powers. In practice, the centre of the pupil is difficult to localise (especially if the patient has dark brown eyes). The measurement is therefore taken from the temporal limbus of one eye to the nasal limbus of the other eye.

One simple method is to sit facing the patient (at the same height) and to place a ruler (with a millimetre scale) across the patient's forehead, so that the rule bisects both pupils. Then direct the patient to look into your right eye (by pointing at your own right eye). Align one line of the ruler with the outer limbus of the patient's *left* eye (close your own left eye to do this, to eliminate possible parallax errors).

Then, without moving the ruler, direct the patient to look into your left eye, and measure the distance to the inner limbus of the patient's *right* eye. The difference between the two measurements is the patient's IPD (for distance viewing) since the eye being measured was effectively looking straight ahead.

Sometimes it is important to measure the IPD at near (for prescribing reading glasses); sit further forward (reading distance) and measure between the outer limbus of one eye and the inner limbus of the other eye while the patient is looking into one of your eyes.

Monocular PD

If a patient has only one eye it is usual to quote the monocular PD, which is the distance from the pupil centre to the midline of the nose. The measurement is taken in a similar way, except that for the right eye, say, two measurements are taken from the midline to the outer limbus, and then from the midline to the inner limbus. The average of these two readings is the monocular PD of the right eye. Monocular PDs are also used in the presence of a marked facial asymmetry.

Potential errors and additional information

Errors are likely to occur if:

- The patient's IPD is vastly different from your own (e.g. young children). This error will increase as the distance between the examiner and the patient decreases.
- The patient does not change fixation from your right to left eye (as this will mean the patient is converging during the measurement).
- The visible corneas are of different sizes. In such a case, measure from the outer limbus of the RE to the inner limbus of the LE, and then from the outer limbus of the LE to the inner limbus of the RE. Average the two readings.
- Do not assume that a ruler is always accurate. Check against a known length (e.g. a steel rule).

Note

- The pupil centre and the visual axis are not usually exactly coincident. This means that IPD is not *exactly* the same as the distance between the visual axes.
- When using a trial frame for near tests, the trial frame can be simply adjusted a few millimetres inwards. When prescribing glasses, this distance can be calculated (or measured) as it depends slightly on the viewing distance, the patient's IPD, and the back vertex distance of the spectacle lenses.

Prescribing glasses for children

Cycloplegia

Accurate subjective refraction depends on the patient being a reasonably reliable observer. Therefore, when refracting children we are more reliant on objective techniques (retinoscopy), and since static retinoscopy depends on accommodation being relaxed for distance viewing, cycloplegia is usually required when refracting young children. There is no definite cut-off age above which cycloplegia is not required – this is a matter of clinical judgement depending on factors other than simply the age of the child.

The drug of choice for cycloplegia is usually either atropine (0.5% or 1%, as ointment or drops) or cyclopentolate (0.5% or 1%). Atropine is typically used to give "full" cycloplegia, in which case the drug is instilled two or three times a day for three days prior to the refraction. It is obvious that even if this is not done at home, the parents must be made aware of possible dangers and side effects. The cycloplegia can last for days afterwards, as can the accompanying mydriasis.

Cyclopentolate is a more convenient drug as it is faster acting, and the effects wear off sooner. The cycloplegia is not as complete as atropine, especially in younger children with significant hypermetropia. However, the difference is less than 0.50 D in many cases, and although full cycloplegia is not produced, the effect is usually sufficient for a reliable refraction. However, the following important points should be noted:

- Cyclopentolate also has potentially hazardous side effects. Cyclopentolate 1% should be used with caution on children below 12 months of age. One drop of 0.5% is a safer option here. For very young or pre-term infants, extreme caution should be exercised.
- The mydriasis occurs on a slightly different time scale to the cycloplegia (try some on your own eye if you don't believe this – typically accommodation is affected first, and some mydriasis remains long after accommodation has returned), and sufficient cycloplegia can be present even though the pupil is still reactive to light. Therefore, do not rely on pupil reactions – get the child to look at your retinoscope and variations in accommodation are easily spotted.

- Children with highly pigmented irides appear to respond less well to cyclopentolate. However, this can often be due to a longer time scale of the onset of maximum action, rather than a vastly reduced effect. Therefore, it may be best to wait longer but always to try cyclopentolate, before resorting to atropine. This simple trial can save the patient many days of blurred vision, and another visit to the clinic.

Once cycloplegia is established, the child can be instructed to look directly at the retinoscope, and the refraction proceeds as normal. It is best to use a trial frame if possible, otherwise hold up spherical lenses. For babies, if the parent holds the child up to look over their shoulder, the patient can be easily approached from behind the parent. Young babies will tend to fixate the retinoscope light if the room is otherwise dark. For older infants, ask the child to sit on their parent's knee. Work as quickly as possible to avoid losing the child's attention. Playing games such as "blowing out the light" can sometimes encourage a youngster to sit still!

Hypermetropia and astigmatism are common in young children, but any refractive error can be present.

If the child has a manifest strabismus, occluding the opposite eye during retinoscopy will ensure that refraction is being measured along the visual axis.

Prescribing

Reasons for prescribing glasses for children can be broadly categorised as:

- to reduce/prevent strabismus in cases of accommodative squint;
- to aid in amblyopia treatment (anisometropia, astigmatism);
- to improve visual acuity in cases of bilateral refractive error (e.g. myopia in a school age child).

Myopia

Remember that for younger (especially pre-school) children, there may be little value in correcting even moderate myopia (above $-3\,\mathrm{D}$ or so, a correction should be considered once the child is mobile). Full or over-treatment of myopia may be justified in the presence of an exodeviation to maintain binocular vision. For school children, educational needs should be considered, and in cases of high refractive errors or poor vision, the teachers should be appraised of any special visual requirements. Advise parents to obtain a spare set of glasses for stronger prescriptions, as they are almost bound to be lost or broken at some stage. Myopia in young children can progress rapidly.

Hypermetropia

Low or moderate hypermetropia is common. The enormous reserves of accommodation of most children mean that refractive errors of the order of 4 D or above may be left without glasses. However, the risk of accommodative strabismus (which must be checked for at distance and near) must not be ignored. In many children, hypermetropia reduces with age. For some, however, glasses may become necessary later in childhood to improve vision (reading) and prevent squint.

For children with esodeviations, the full hypermetropic correction may be required to maintain, or establish binocular vision. In some cases, this can be seen as a diagnostic trial.

Astigmatism

Low to moderate astigmatism is not uncommon in children. The risk of meridional amblyopia increases in cases with significant astigmatism (2 D or more) at age 2 years and above. Astigmatism should be corrected where it is considered that a risk of amblyopia exists, or to improve vision (e.g. at school). Significant astigmatism will reduce both near and distance VA.

Anisometropia

Studies have shown that anisometropia can come and go, and even reverse in young children. Anisometropic corrections should be tried in children with amblyopia, or who are at risk of amblyopia. The highest risk occurs when one eye is nearly emmetropic and the opposite eye has high myopia – luckily such cases are rare. Significant hypermetropia of one eye is the next highest risk, but any child with more than 0.50 D difference between the eyes should be considered at potential risk of developing amblyopia.

If glasses are prescribed, the full correction need not be given, so long as the anisometropia is corrected: in other words, if the refraction is RE +2.00 DS LE +4.0 DS, a prescription of RE plano LE +2.00 DS would correct the anisometropia. For some children with anisometropic amblyopia, glasses alone may bring the vision up before resorting to occlusion therapy.

216

There is some debate as to the underlying cause of anisometropia, and the cause and effect relationship with amblyopia is by no means clear in all cases.

Strabismus

The relationship between vergence and accommodation means that full correction of hypermetropia will usually reduce esodeviations. Do not be overly concerned if a pre-school child has reduced distance vision in their full correction – the more important consideration is stable binocular vision. If there are worries about distinguishing between amblyopia and the over-correction of hypermetropia, these are resolved by testing visual acuity with a reduced prescription in the trial frame, by holding minus lenses over the glasses, or with the pinhole in older children.

Exodeviations can sometimes be reduced or controlled by giving minus lenses. This therapy is limited by the importance of good near vision.

In some cases of anisometropia, one eye is easily suppressed, and a squint becomes manifest unless the spectacle correction is worn.

Aphakia

Cycloplegia is obviously not required here. However, the difficulties include:

- The power of the convex lenses means that glasses are thick, heavy, unsightly, and difficult to fit. The spectacle lens/eye combination is not ideal optically due to aberrations. Aspheric spectacle lens designs go some way to reducing these problems.
- For young children full-time wear of aphakic spectacles is almost impossible to achieve. Contact lenses present a better optical situation, and present one of the few instances where the risks of contact lens wear in children are outweighed by the potential benefits.
- In unilateral aphakia, the amblyopia risk is very high. Spectacles are not usually considered an option due to the enormous difference in refractive power of the eyes. Such cases are better treated using a contact lens, or intra-ocular lens.

Notes

- Specify plastics or safety lenses for children to reduce the risk from splinters of broken glass.

217

- Many children will throw their glasses off. If a child is reluctant to wear a new hypermetropic prescription, it may be worth reducing the lens power if this can be done without inducing strabismus. Some practitioners advocate a short course of atropinisation so that vision is clearer with the glasses on.
- Refractive errors can change rapidly in childhood – regular refractions may be required, sometimes as often as once every six to eight weeks for an aphakic baby, every three to six months for a young infant.
- High refractive errors that do not "emmetropise" may indicate an underlying pathology.

Contact lens fitting

Contact lenses (CLs) can be categorised by their type, and the material from which they are made:

- Rigid corneal lenses: hard (daily wear) or gas permeable (daily wear or extended wear).
- Soft lenses: hydrogels (daily wear, extended wear, disposables) or silicone.
- Scleral lenses (usually PMMA, gas permeable types are becoming more widely available).

The uses of CLs include:

- Refractive correction.
- To protect the cornea (bandage lens).
- To improve cosmesis of an unsightly eye.
- As part of a drug delivery system (e.g. collagen shields).
- As part of orthoptic treatment (e.g. occlusion using a high powered or opaque lens).

A detailed description of CL fitting is beyond the scope of this work, and several excellent texts are available. The steps in fitting contact lenses are briefly described.

Patient selection

CL wear is not as easy as it initially appears, and the ideal patient would be a responsible, intelligent adult who is highly motivated to succeed! Young children do not make good patients unless the parents are willing to assume a large degree of responsibility for inserting, removing, and caring for the contact lenses. Extended wear should be avoided unless necessary, especially for children, due to the increased risk of corneal infection.

Patients with significant refractive errors (the improvement in vision for a high myope, or an aphake can be dramatic), keratoconus, or patients in need of cosmetic lenses are often willing to put up with the additional expense and drawbacks of contact lenses.

Lens selection

The pros and cons of different lens types, such as the Table below, can aid in lens selection.

Type of lens	Pros	Cons
Hard (PMMA) corneal lenses	Cheap	Need to be fitted loose to ensure adequate tear exchange
	Durable	Initially uncomfortable
	Well tolerated once the initial discomfort is past	Limited wearing times
Scleral lenses	Many cases which are otherwise impossible to fit can be fitted	Limited wearing time due to poor oxygen supply to cornea
	Unsightly eyes can be hidden	Expensive and time consuming to fit
	Ptosis support possible	
	Virtually any refractive error (including advanced keratoconus) can be fitted	
Rigid gas permeable lenses	Adequate oxygen supply to cornea may be achieved	More expensive than hard lenses
	Long wearing times possible	Lens spoilation and breakage may limit life
	Few after-care problems	Expensive solutions often required
Soft (hydrophilic) lenses	Little or no initial discomfort	Often abused by patients
	Extended wear may be possible	After-care expensive
	Children can usually tolerate soft lenses	Increased risk of infection
		Limited lens life
		Lens deposits may give rise to problems
Silicon rubber lenses	Excellent gas permeability	Poor (high) wetting angle means that lenses "stick" to eye, and may be difficult to remove
	Extended wear possible	May be uncomfortable
	The lens of choice for some aphakic infants (as silicon lenses do not easily fall out of the eye)	Expensive

The patient should have a full examination of the anterior eye and eye lids to check for infections, irregularities, tear quality etc.

The corneal shape is measured using a keratometer or corneal topographer, and a trial contact lens is inserted. The power of this lens should be as close as possible to ideal, and can be approximated from the formula: $F_c = F_s / (1 - d \cdot F_s)$ where F_c = contact lens power, F_s = spectacle lens power and d = the back vertex distance of the spectacle lens. Therefore, a myopic spectacle wearer will require less power in their contact lens than the spectacle lens.

After the initial lacrimation has subsided, the position of the lens is checked and the patient can be left to allow the lens to settle.

The fit of a rigid lens is initially checked using fluorescein and a blue lamp with a magnifier to allow the lens to be easily seen (Burton lamp). Closer inspection is made using a slit lamp, and the ideal lens will:

- fit more or less centrally on the cornea so that the pupil is covered by the optic of the lens;
- have sufficient edge lift to allow a good exchange of tears;
- follow the corneal contour in such a way that the lens is neither too tight nor loose a fit.

The effect of blinking on lens position and movement is noted. If the lens moves excessively or insufficiently, the fit should be altered. Ideally, the lens will move by between 1 and 3 mm, and will quickly recentre after a blink.

For a soft lens, fluorescein should not be used as it will not easily wash out of the lens, and the fit is assessed by observing lens position and movement, and by assessing the quality of vision before and after blinking.

Over-refraction should then be carried out to work out the power required. The final lens is ordered, and when it arrives from the manufacturer, must be tried in the eye before the patient leaves, as some change of fit can be expected if the trial and final lens have different powers.

Contact lens wear is normally limited to 2–4 hours on the first day for rigid lenses (4–6 hours for soft lenses) and is gradually increased up to a maximum period, which depends on the lens type, the physiologic response of the eye, and the needs of the patient.

Notes

- All contact lenses can be expected to be initially slightly uncomfortable. Soft lenses are usually the most comfortable, and a gas permeable lens may produce a sensation similar to an eyelash in the eye initially. This feeling should subside. Always check for trapped particles under the lens if the patient has a strong response. One problem with hard (PMMA) lenses over the long term is desensitisation of the cornea, caused by reduced oxygen supply and habituation. Such cases can present with foreign body tracks in the corneal epithelium, the patient being completely unaware of any problem.

221

- The lens fit, power, design, and material will determine how much gas exchange takes place. The individual needs of the patient and their environment may necessitate a highly gas permeable design, and epithelial or mild corneal oedema is strongly suggestive of such a need.
- Be aware of the risks of contact lens wear, and discontinue lens wear in the presence of conjunctivitis, infective blepharitis, or corneal irregularity.
- Advise patients to carry a spare pair of glasses and their contact lens case so they can remove the lenses at any time.

Index